Dopa_____

How Technology Is Creating a Dystopian World

(Helping You Become More Effective in Your Everyday Living)

By Reggie Lashley

Published By **Ryan Princeton**

Reggie Lashley

Dopamine: How Technology Is Creating a Dystopian World (Helping You Become More Effective in Your Everyday Living)

ISBN   978-1-77485-468-6

Legal & Disclaimer

The information contained in this ebook is not designed to replace or take the place of any form of medicine or professional medical advice. The information in this ebook has been provided for educational & entertainment purposes only.

The information contained in this book has been compiled from sources deemed reliable, and it is accurate to the best of the Author's knowledge; however, the Author cannot guarantee its accuracy and validity and cannot be held liable for any errors or omissions. Changes are periodically made to this book. You must consult your doctor or get professional medical advice before using any of the suggested remedies, techniques, or information in this book.

Upon using the information contained in this book, you agree to hold harmless the Author from and against any damages, costs, and expenses, including any legal fees potentially resulting from the application of any of the information provided by this guide. This disclaimer applies to any damages or injury caused by the use and application, whether directly or indirectly, of any advice or information presented, whether for breach of contract, tort, negligence, personal injury, criminal intent, or under any other cause of action.

You agree to accept all risks of using the information presented inside this book. You need to consult a professional medical practitioner in order to ensure you are both able and healthy enough to participate in this program.

TABLE OF CONTENTS

Introduction... 1

chapter 1: explains what is dopamine?.... 3

chapter 2: negativity and us.................. 20

chapter 3: the negativity bias................. 71

chapter 4: comprehensive explanation of dopamine... 109

chapter 5: benefits of meditative, yoga, and other activities during a dopamine fast 121

chapter 6: what are the do's and don'ts of dopamine fasting 125

chapter 7: dopamine fast challenge 130

chapter 8: how to stay motivated and keep from stopping your dopamine quickly . 135

chapter 9: definition of negativity........ 139

conclusion.. 183

Introduction

Our brain is an incredible feat. It's an organ that is responsible for every action both the outside and inside within the human body. When it comes to lifting the hand, or breathing in, your brain is a key component in every single one of these activities. In terms of feelings or moods, brain is the most powerful medicine. The release of chemical substances within the human body regulates the intensity of these emotions that people go through. One of these chemicals is known as Dopamine. The chemical is helpful in altering and controlling behaviours. Dopamine release in the body leads to the individual feeling stimulated and feeling a sense of satisfaction.

As we age the levels of dopamine in the body change with time. For instance, it's very low in adolescents, which is not surprising. Dopamine is a chemical that is released by the body, and is often referred to as the natural mood-enhancing drug. The decrease in levels of dopamine could cause a decrease in motivation, inability to concentrate on tasks, fatigue, and inability to complete anything.

In keeping that all in mind, the most effective solutions to this problem could be Dopamine Fasting. This technique is believed to aid people in creating an ongoing routine however, it also assists to stay organized and steers the life of a person towards an organized and clear path.

Chapter 1: Explains What Is Dopamine?

Dopamine is the reason for the pleasure that you feel when engaging in pleasurable pursuits like sexual activity, surfing social media and get in love, get to know new people, have a good time with friends e.t.c

Dopamine induces a sense of enthusiasm, motivation, and hunger. A few of the popular stimulants of dopamine is alcohol and alcohol, both of which can be addictive.

It is essential that everyone to have a healthy supply of dopamine. A lack of it could cause mood swings, Parkinson's disease and depression.

Dopamine's functions

Dopamine enhances learning as well as attention and memory

* Dopamine improves ability to think critically

* Dopamine boosts motivation when performing tasks.

* Dopamine can help with depression.

How Dopamine Works

Dopamine's main function allows signals from one neuron to the next to flow through synapses. Further, the neurons make use of dopamine, and the results can differ dependent on the kind of neurons involved, as well as the different receptors make use of dopamine for connecting the neurons.

Dopamine was a key component in the transmission of signals. At first, scientists believed it was connected to the pleasure. People suffering from depression are more likely to have lower levels of dopamine in their brains, which led researchers to conclude that the low dopamine levels made them less satisfied.

The idea is still bouncing around across popular media since it is believed to be relevant. But by the end of the 1980s, scientific research had ruled out the idea. Research has shown that animals whose dopamine neurons were killed through drugs still enjoyed the sugar taste when it was squeezed in their mouths. However, they didn't seek out another type of sugar.

Dopamine is not a source of pleasure, it does affect the pleasure that the brain produces. However, the method by which it does this differs from opinions. One theory is that the main impact of dopamine is that it can boost pleasure to the point that the brain is conditioned to anticipate this result of the actions. Examining gamblers, for instance, revealed that the brain is able to produce more dopamine than it does when winning. It's like the chemical is urging them to be successful each time.

Another theory is that dopamine simply aids the brain to become more engaged and makes the body feel more powerful enough to pull the lever up often.

Dopamine and addiction

Dopamine is the primary driver that drives your desires and need. It is the reason why you desire what you desire. This is the basis component of what you want.

If you complete something that feels great, there is a good likelihood that you'll repeat it again , but if it's wasn't as rewarding, we won't be driven to do it again because it's like a punishment.

The brain part that produces the pleasant feeling in our brains is called dopamine. It triggers a feeling of need in us. And because we desire this wonderful feeling, we create an habit of doing things that release dopamine production in the brain. In the course of time the normal doesn't stimulate it, which means there's a need to boost the dose or seek it out in another way. That's when the sex, drugs, and alcohol addictions develop.

Dopamine and reward

Dopamine is a reward when we perform tasks which require an enormous amount of effort, such as the time we get food after battling for it, or when we triumph in a difficult competition after having lost hope.

The reason why we feel a pleasant feeling that follows this achievement is that it increases our security.

The only way to trigger dopamine is when you get unexpected rewards. When you've been working hard for something and then find yourself rewarded even though your chances of getting it are slim. If you receive an unexpected and overwhelming reward, you are overwhelmed with dopamine. For example, you're hoping to earn $40 at the conclusion of a contract , only to receive a cash reward of $60. The surprise reward causes dopamine.

If we are suddenly the reward of something that is higher than the expectations of others, it makes us feel so great. When we are used to receiving $60 in the same contract, the dopamine levels drop. The reason is that we did not get what we expected.

How businesses and brands use dopamine to make money

Businesses and big brands spend millions of dollars in research to figure the most effective methods for keeping their clients to purchase more products.

A lot of people are spending hours that could be spent doing something productive on social media. Think about the amount of hours you are seated and scroll through your social media accounts every day, or browsing the web. The time you spend on social media could be better used to do something productive but your brain needs social media more since it's designed to keep you hooked for the overwhelming feeling it gives you.

The internet and a majority of social media sites use an algorithm that keeps users on their site for a long time like, Twitter. You're looking to read one tweet, but you realize that there's an a million others you must check out, and because it was enjoyable and you want to check for the next one. The initial goal was to check out only one tweet. This continues until you've read more than 100 tweets.

It is also apparent when playing video games. Games that use levels and ranking system, so that when you've completed a stage in the game you go to the next stage and each stage gives you a shot of dopamine.

The dopamine reward system is present in porn alcohol, and a lot of other things which provide instant gratification.

Dopamine is more influential on our behavior than any other instrument. Everyone is affected by it. That's why people are spending more time with digital content rather than living the life they wish to live.

How do you control dopamine levels

Dopamine Detoxation to increase your reward levels

Dopamine fasting rids your body of everything that can increase your levels of dopamine. Drugs, destructive habits junk food, junk food as well as social media and many other things that can make you excited and give you a huge joy.

In our daily lives, we might be tempted to chase dopamine and it can become harmful. Dopamine triggers are best found with regard to rewards and unanticipated and therefore, when we actively seek the pleasure of dopamine us, we've created a harmful dependence to the neurotransmitter.

The amount of time you devote to on the internet when you are working on a crucial task to finish. Dopamine urges you to binge go back to the TV or browse more when you ought to be working on that office project you've put off for days.

Dopamine-driven fasting is crucial for the development of your resistance to the temptation. It offers you a better sense that you are in control of your behavior and alters the way you interact to dopamine.

Discipline

The biggest challenge we'll face when pursuing the life we've always wanted is discipline. As we strive to achieve our objectives

Dopamine-inducing actions will keep us from attaining the objectives we have set.

Discipline can be very difficult. Most of the time we'll be demotivated. Sometimes, it can trigger feelings of anger, loneliness, frustration and regret, as well as anxiety, fear, or anxiety within our mind. The feelings can be painful and hurtful. The idea of avoiding the task may appear to be the most sensible choice.

When we pursue our goals, with discipline, we discover the purpose of our lives, but when we stay clear of uncomfortable emotions, how can we discover our comfort? The process of pursuing your goal is gruellingly difficult and incredibly rewarding. This is the difference that separates winners from the losers. The losers go for the safe way and stay clear of the discomfort associated with chase purposes. Winners embrace it. As said by Michael Jordan, I have missed over 9000 shots over my entire career. I've lost almost 300 games. In 26 occasions, I've tasked to make the shot that won but failed. I've failed over and over in my entire life. This is the reason I am successful.

Many people fail to pursue their goals because of the cost that is involved. They delay or avoid the issue. They may even use alcohol and drugs to lessen their bodies to discomfort. These painful experiences allow us to develop mentally, emotionally and spiritually. If we wish to improve and be successful then we need to learn to accept pain and discomfort instead of avoiding them.

To be able to achieve the most amazing accomplishments, we have to master the art of discipline to achieve our goals. There are two steps to mastering discipline.

Acceptance of the responsibility

To be disciplined We must first recognize our own shortcomings. It is important to learn to accept the responsibility of pursuing our goals. We need to realize that we're in control of our lives and where we'll get to is the consequence the actions we take and actions.

No one will accomplish our objectives on our behalf. What happens to your life out is your own responsibility. Inventing excuses or blame someone else for your problems won't get you anywhere and can only hinder your progress.

It is also important to be accountable for our feelings. Our happiness, sadness and suffering do not rest with others. It is in our own control. Once we take responsibility for our actions decisions, and emotions and feelings, we're prepared to develop.

A painful determination to pursue

We must take a decision to follow our mission regardless of the cost. We have to confront the issues we've been trying to avoid. We've fully taken responsibility for our decision to take action, and there's no excuses. The first step is to build positive habits slowly and continuously.

It won't be easy and you'll be demotivated at times however, you have to keep going with a lot of pain. You've got your own willpower to depend on. It's a gradual change between "I will write an article for my forthcoming manuscript whenever I am motivated to write this" to"I have completed an entire chapter for my forthcoming manuscript every night since I must".

A chapter every evening is less effort and if you do it, you'll end up with an entirely completed manuscript within a certain time.

It would be impossible in the absence of motivation.

Every habit is maintained and enriched by the habit of writing, reading or even walking. Sit still and avoid walking for a week and observe the results. Whatever you're trying to establish as your routine a habit, you must practice it consistently. There is nothing more important than that.

Benefits of fasting with dopamine

* More Productivity

* Focused on

* Controlled actions and decisions

* Fewer distractions

• Replace harmful behaviors with healthier ones, which will improve your quality of life.

How do you carry out dopamine elimination

The first step to carry out the dopamine rush is to identify the temptations and instant gratifications you'd like to rid yourself of, such as eating unhealthy foods, social networks intake porn, video games, t.v and etcetera.

Next, you must formulate an action plan that is realistic. It could be that you cut down on your consumption of sugary drinks by reducing your intake from 5 times per day to just 2 times per day or limit your time on social media from unlimited hours to two minutes per day. This seems more achievable and feasible since the idea of cutting completely off social media is almost impossible. Your brain is used to this, and it could take time to adapt. It is recommended to reduce gradually the habit until you're able to eliminate it completely.

You must be accountable to someone or something. When you're accountable to something or someone will increase the likelihood of completing on your goals. You could make yourself accountable for someone else, using a notepad, a journal or a tracker app for your habits. Lack of accountability causes your focus wane.

Next step would be to simply begin. At first it's going to be tough. If you're determined then you'll begin seeing the rewards quickly.

How to Increase Naturally Dopamine levels inside the brain

Meditation is a process of developing the mind and fostering awareness of the mind. Meditation helps us gain control over our thoughts, energy and feelings.

When we practice meditation it is a time to dedicate our time and energy to be conscious. Through meditation, we decide to be aware of our thoughts.

How do you meditate?

Sit comfortably and be focused in your breathing. Try to block out thoughts that come through the corners of your brain. The mind functions like an muscle. The more you work it to strengthen it, the stronger it becomes. There are a myriad of distractions, in the form of thoughts and smells, memories, and even sensations. Take note of them and return to your breath.

Be careful not to get carried by thoughts. Keep your attention upon your breathing. Breathe deeply in and out. When you go and you notice it, smile and keep meditating. The present moment should be the sole thing you are able to live in. Every day, you should practice for ten to fifteen minutes, or longer.

1. Exercise

Studies have proven that exercise boosts our mood. Exercise can increase levels of dopamine, which increases our attention, memory as well as problem-solving and memory.

It's been demonstrated in a variety of studies that exercise regularly is a remedy for anxiety and depression. Exercise can improve the health of patients suffering from mental illness.

Activities like walking, running or biking, yoga, swimming and lifting weights have an great benefits to our physical and mental well-being.

1. Enjoy delicious food

Beans blueberries, walnuts, walnuts, soybeans are loaded with proteins and can increase levels of dopamine within the body.

Eliminate processed, sugary and carbonated foods.

1. Sleep enough

Achieving 7-9 hours of rest each day boosts your overall mood, reduces stress levels and helps keep your energy levels up.

Dopamine is released by the body at night prior to bed and also in the morning, after you get up. Sleeping enough helps maintain your levels of dopamine.

Insufficient sleep makes your body slow, clogged and inactive.

1. Sunlight exposure

A lack of exposure to sunlight has been associated with low levels of neurotransmitters, such as dopamine. Exposure to sunlight can raise dopamine levels in the body.

The study shows that those who were exposed to more sunlight had higher levels of dopamine receptors.

Dopamine levels increase in the sun. in the body. However, excessive exposure to sunlight may cause harm to the body.

How do you optimize dopamine levels to be successful?

Dopamine is connected directly to your Prefrontal Cortex (PFC), that makes the decisions. (More than the other brain part The "you" part is your PFC.)

Dopamine is connected to the PFC through the mesocortical pathway. Dopamine that is an emotion and motivation system is in sync and with cortical (and limbic) systems. The emotional system as well as the logic system function as two different sides of a coin in the PFC.

You can manage your motivation if you can manage your dopamine system.

If most people focus on the same objective their brains release a significant quantity of dopamine.

It's as pleasurable for them as they are playing.

Imagine feeling the same satisfaction when you sit in front of your computer's screen and typing away just like eating the perfect Belgian waffle by Nutella and your favourite coffee that is made to perfection.

Certain people are able to develop their brains in an approach that they release enormous amounts of dopamine through pursuing a goal.

Why?

It's because of the brain mechanism that makes sure that the release of dopamine from"the "expectancy of the reward" is higher over the amount of reward.

This push is generated by dopamine, which helps get the desired reward.

If you asked those who are hard-working and enjoy their own way, you'd probably hear some very insightful phrases, but not the main motive behind it. To find the truth it is necessary to pose the question not directly to the person , but rather at their mind.

Since the dopamine and PFC centers within the brain connected through the mesocortical pathway the way you approach the particular task can affect the amount of dopamine released, and how much you're motivated to accomplish the task.

How do you train your brain to create more dopamine, thus motivating you to take on more?

* Establish goals. The system is not effective without a predetermined reward to be earned. (Use individual notes on annual or 5-year goals, such.)

* Design Triggers. You need to communicate to your brain that work is about to begin and what's to come in the future. (Visually be surrounded by visual reminders to remember your objectives and tasks, to-do lists as well as schedules and so on.)

Goals must be accompanied by rewards. (Just be sure that you know the existence of rewards.) The goals you set, like being fit or achieving the first a thousand paying customers typically are worthwhile and rewarding by themselves However, you must add an additional reward.

* Add a hint of surprise. Dopamine release increases when reward uncertainty is present. When rewards occur 50 percent of the time instead of 100 percent all the time the release of dopamine increases by a factor of two! If you're not convinced, head to the casino and look at the crowd. The most effective way to achieve this is to go into the field that you're not familiar with, and then to change the kinds of objectives and tasks you assign yourself to ensure the sake of novelty.

Chapter 2: Negativity And Us

The disorders associated with depression and anxiety typically have a high percentage that is characterized by catastrophic thoughts.

Patients are more likely to imagine, think about and believe in the worst possible outcomes in their struggles and fears, frequently fantasizing about dramatic scenarios which rarely happen for them or anyone else.

Let's begin with a few examples that illustrate this characteristic very well:

A person suffering from panic disorder frequently believes that their heart beats that pound result in an attack of the heart, or that their headaches could be the first sign of stroke.

* A person with generalized anxiety disorder speaks via phone with his wife. She informs him that he's going to travel on the bus with his children and he is worried that one of them might fall into the wheels of the bus and die.

* A person who is depressed thinks that his family doesn't believe in him and thinks that within a couple of years, he'll become lonely, abandoned and dying in a public hospital for homeless persons.

These are but a few examples that illustrate the typical situation of catastrophism. It is not only due to the dramatic scenario that the patient is able to imagine in his head however, it is also since the fearful event has never occurred to him, and the odds for it occurring are tiny. But, the patient cannot not think about it, and the subsequent suffering it results in.

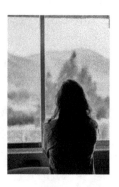

Let's just assume that a person believes or believes in numerous instances of a negative event that isn't happening. Numerous times they're incorrect, yet because of reasons that are beyond their control they do not take into consideration the evidence that proves the event they're afraid of doesn't occur. So, they continue thinking about tragic scenarios within their heads.

It's like we get up each morning thinking that when we open the window, we'll be able to see a stunning landscape of mountains and sea and mountains, but instead, we see a dark lung that is growing. Although today, and every morning before I've seen the same lung that is growing but it doesn't matter. I will wake up on the next day with the hope that the stunning scenery will be revealed before me. Absurd, right?

This is how absurd it is to us, that each day we are afflicted with fears of things that haven't happened. Of course it's easier to recognize the absurdity of positive facts than an unfavourable one, and something that has to do with the origins and the nature of the catastrophic mindset.

In the beginning million in years of development have created permanent impressions on our brains including an increase in the capacity to deal to uncertainty, fear and uncertainty. Imagine an animal living in a primitive setting that is a natural setting like a forest or a jungle. There is a distinctive sound from the trees.

A defensive response like fear can help your survival event of predators' possible presence. I've mentioned this scenario previously. In contrast the "upbeat" response such as not alerting yourself can cause death.

In the environment of the past which has existed throughout thousands of years of development of life. Fear has been proven to be an essential adaptation that it will not survive. Therefore, it is evident that we today have an greater capacity to react defensively to uncertain situations. In the present, the fear reaction is triggered by a number of responses and levels, one of which is the cognitive. This is what causes catastrophism.

It is the result of the cognitive manifestation of an evolved facilitated tendency. This is because considering the most dangerous potential outcomes helps us adapt to a more objectively hostile environment, in which dangers were more common than the modern environment.

However being optimistic and positive could be a danger of not being able to react quickly to threats that, if it was real could cause us to be thrown from our evolutionary lineage. The way we think about this has evolved in the modern and civilized environment where the majority of people live, but primitive reactions remain in our brains' deepest regions and brains, remnants of our past.

The previous thesis partially addresses the issue of catastrophism as a mental way of thinking. Although it's real that it offers us an important insight into why we respond easily to fears and panic to uncertain situations, and why optimism isn't instinctual and easy for us?

However it remains open to the problem of why some are prone to destructive thinking that causes stress, or as well as the formation of mental disorders , while others are successful in conquering the primitive mind within us.

Also, why in the realm of catastrophic thinking does it become regular or intense and lasts for a long time for some people, while it is intermittent, mild and brief in others? Like most times there is no one solution to this issue.

Research in neuroscience has revealed that individuals have differences caused by hereditary causes. In the end, all organs in the body have their own genetic factory mark. The brain is not required to be an one of them. While this is interesting however, it is far beyond the goals of this chapter.

Reacting to fear requires learning. While as an emotional response it is instinctual however, we are taught how to respond to it. Experiences of stress in the beginning contribute to the vulnerability in the psychological system. Therefore, having extremely traumatized childhood experiences, or being within an emotional unstable environment in the early years makes the body with a higher risk of shoot, and with greater in frequency and intensity.

In some way, the early years are marked by an impression when we've had to endure difficult experiences, we are given the message that "our surroundings are dangerous, hostile, and consequently, it is essential to always be prepared to defend ourselves" and we develop a habit of thinking about catastrophe, as during our first few years we've proven that "it is best to always be ready."

Another crucial aspect in sustaining the frightful thoughts is the actions we take when these thoughts arise. This is, after the terrifying thoughts are surfacing in our mind, and we begin to feel worried What do we do? What should we tell ourselves? How can we handle these issues? This issue is particularly relevant to the psychology clinic since they are one of the avenues of our ability to lessen the impact of this issue.

In certain situations individuals who experience the thought of a catastrophic event not only responds to it emotionally in an uncontrollable way but also utters or engages in behaviors that are designed to reduce anxiety, without questioning the validity of the thought. They are in the belief that they believe that what they are thinking is true simply because they perceive that their thoughts have their own weight, just like factual evidence. This is a mistake.

The fact that I have a mental image constantly in my head isn't a guarantee that the truth depicted by the image objectively more likely. The most striking instances is seen in patients with health anxiety. They have a mild abdominal pain think they are suffering from an infected tumor.

The thought of the tumor, and imagining the treatment and diagnosis of a disease like cancer doesn't increase the chance of suffering. Most of the time, because of an unfounded fear the patients will visit their doctor for assurance in the absence of any evidence. This is easy since they suffer from stomach indigestion, information that they already knew since they've suffered through this experience numerous times.

In this manner, unneeded trips to the physician transform into reinsurance behavior that hinders an easy verification process which, in the long time, could result in the elimination of anxiety. The things we thought were true simply do not occur. The issue is made worse due to the fact that, even though theories aren't true but it is true that the frequency we consider these ideas makes them appear to be to be more probable which is referred to as subjective or heuristic probability.

Our brains estimate the likelihood of an event by using two kinds of analysis. The first follows rational and logical guidelines, like that derived from a statistical study that suggests that flying is the most secure method of transportation of all.

There is an estimate of the probabilities that is based on how many times we've thought about an occurrence. The more often we think about it and the more likely it is that we are convinced of it regardless of our actual information. Because of this, people with a fear believe that their plane will crash as they've been thinking about it numerous times.

This is also the reason why the person in our earlier example, who had health anxiety, believes the person is extremely likely to develop cancer no more and more than simply because she often thinks about it.

This is known as subjective or heuristic probability an approach that can be summarized by saying that at times when we consider some thing, we end up not knowing if it is actually true and how much of it is something we've created it.

For some individuals these factors are convergent more than other people, but with the exact same pattern, which results in the fear response and its cognitional equivalent, the catastrophic thought being expressed with greater frequency in intensity, duration, and intensity.

If we all have an evolutionary and biologically facilitated tendency to be anxious however, we have individual differences in what we inherit as well as in the way we were taught in the crucial period of our childhood, and in the way we handle terrifying thoughts once they are presented.

Why do we sigh? What does it have to do with Stress?

The act can have a touch of romantic in the way it is performed, like with this exhalation, we release our sadness, our regret of longing or the desire to be loved. Sighing for many is another language that expresses affection and can be poetically described as the soul's cry. But is there any truth in the whole thing?

In reality, very little. But there is one thing is essential to be clear about: sighing can be an important physiological process. It is crucial for lung health and for emotional health. In addition the brain is dependent on it to the point where neurologists have defined this process to be"the "mental reset" button.

Find out more below.

"Our crying is an insignificant thing. Sighs are just a tiny item... But even for such little things, we and you will be dead". Emily Dickinson. Emily Dickinson

Why do we sigh?

Consider taking a moment to answer the following questions: how often per day do you think about sighing? Do you happen to be one of those who sighs every two to three minutes? It's not just like the typical questions that children everywhere have, it is not forgotten that something as regular everyday as sighing vital to many living things"integral health.

Since not just humans do it But when we examine our pets, it is possible to be able to see how our dogs and cats perform it. Are they also able to get in love, or do they feel sad or angry? We don't know for sure but what we recognize is the fact that this method is crucial to maintain the health of your lung.

Additionally, if we don't take these inhalations regularly all day long, we'll be dead.

The sighs, a crucial reflection

"Sigh and live. It sounds like a line that comes from a commercial however, it's not. We now understand this mechanism in greater detail and to the point where research published in

Nature describes it as a crucial reflection. We've discovered that there are two tiny types of nerve cells inside the brain stem, which control the process.

The cell's principal function is to control breathing, sleep and the heartbeat. We now know that it also triggers the Sigh mechanism.

Why is that? If we think about the reason we feel like we're groaning and sigh, the answer is easy that we want to prevent the alveoli from bursting. There are occasions when these tiny sacs which are the lungs' and regulate the exchange of carbon dioxide and oxygen become stuck.

The reason for the sigh is to cause the collapsed alveoli to be filled by a greater amount of air than normal to activate its function.

If we didn't take action, we'd begin to experience lung failure.

The scientist behind this research Professor Dr. Jack Feldman, professor of neurobiology at the University of Los Angeles School of Medicine is able to tell us something equally fascinating. The brain triggers various breathing patterns thanks to neuropeptides which regulate breathing in normal situations such as coughing, yawning, crying, and laughing.

Sighs are also controlled by only 200 neurons, a extremely small number of nerve cells that are capable of fulfilling our vital task.

When you're stressedout, do you feel more stressed?

We were able to feel sighs recently, when they were just a few deep breaths that are associated with emotional pain and sadness. We now know that your job is to fill the alveolis with air. However, is that their sole function? Actually, they perform a lot more for us.

Sighs are more frequent when we are suffering from stress , and can even be caused by some psychiatric disorders: schizophrenia, bipolar disorder and psychosis. In any situation where our mood is at extreme intensity, sighs be heard. They are a way to ease tension and release the stress that our body and mind are exposed to.

However studies like ones conducted in the University of Leuven, in Belgium provide us with another aspect. When asked the reason we sigh it is important to provide a different reason: to restore equilibrium within the brain. It's as if you reset your mind, as if the brain is bringing oxygen in to conceal the negative.

This is the reason we can't not help but sigh long when we're overwhelmed with anger or sadness, despair or even boredom. Sighs don't just stretch the pulmonary alveoli but also fills the air chambers. In doing this it creates a sense of mental relief can also be felt as we get oxygenated and we feel calm and the entire body recovers its homeostasis.

How do Negativity and Constant complaining affect our brains?

One person is matched with another. In just five minutes, the one is awestruck and speechless while hearing his friend's complaints. The complaints are about his siblings, parents and the absence of work as well as the absence of an associate, the horrible health care system, the absence of understanding by his neighbours, and inexplicably arbitrary policies of the government.

There are certain situations in life that are sure to cause us to complain, as a natural response to relieve tensions that have been accumulated from the event. The loss of a beloved family member, or being laid off because of a cut in staff divorce, a separation or grave illness are difficult events for which complaining will bring us closer.

"He was one who was a person who enjoyed the plight of his life and was more likely to complain than alter it." - John Katzenbach

Some people do complain about their food. In addition, they believe that all "good people" all over the world have to hear the petty complaints since, if they didn't they'd be proving that they're not sensitive or self-centered.

Modern complaints

The modern world isn't an easy task. Everyday, we are bombarded with stories, which are often painful or stressful. In addition, we have to endure angry bosses or bounced employees and the personal issues that we face including illness, loss and a myriad of circumstances that can end up acrid.

When faced with a situation like this there are two options: examine each scenario, find the most effective way to deal with it or resist and accept the perspective of the complainer. The problem with the second option is that it can become an habit that reduces our possibilities and creates an attitude of negativity in the people who are around us.

It is possible to believe it's a type of catharsis when we are in the midst of stress, and it can, in some instances serve this purpose. However, without us being aware of it, our complaint could become a habit we repeat in a loop and, over time, will become the standard response to problems.

Consequences of our brain

Based on research conducted by neuroscientists from various fields the frequency and intensity of our emotions will vary will depend on whether the brain undergoes major changes. This is because in this state of perpetual frustration and powerlessness the brain releases hormones like cortisol, norepinephrine, and adrenaline which ultimately can alter how it functions. the organ.

Researchers have suggested that repeated exposure to the problem erodes or even eliminates the neural connections in the brain's hippocampus. This is the specific part responsible for coming up with solutions to the problems that plague us.

Insistence on complaining is a means to negatively impose our beliefs on ourselves, which leads to disdain in others and ultimately ends with a decline in the quality of our family, relationship or workplace relationships. It's a sign of dependence and, consequently in a state of immaturity and naiveté in the face of challenges.

The Negative Effect of Thinking, and the Decline in Cognitive Function: wear and tear of our Brain

Cognitive decline and negative thinking are closely linked. A factor that can raise, according to various studies, the likelihood of suffering from memory loss attention, language or orientation issues in older years is to be a victim of those mental habits where negativity persists and is chronic. It is a fact that we must think about and keep in mind.

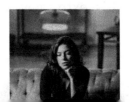

We are aware of it, the majority of us know that the things we think we like favors or hampers our quality of life. Furthermore, it's not just the perception we give to what is around us, or the events that occur to improve our health or to increase suffering. It's also our emotions and emotions that influence the brain and, consequently, many of the neurochemical processes.

It is impossible to overlook, for instance the effects that continuous stress can have on certain areas, such as the hippocampus the brain region that is associated with memory. When we are in a state of psychological stress, where anxiety is never-ending and negative thoughts or anxiety are prevalent, the creation the development of neuronal cells is severely reduced. This means that over time it will not just become more difficult to learn new things and also the link between nerve cells diminishes in quality.

Cognitive decline and negative thinking: how do they relate?

We all have moments where worry is a constant companion, as a storm clouds in the summertime. It's extremely stressful, but it doesn't last for long. Things change quickly and we come up with strategies to deal with these issues and then we return to peace and stability. Being in these situations is normal and nothing can affect the neurological system.

Furthermore, the simple necessity of looking for solutions, being creative and use methods to tackle problems brings back the health of our brains: we increase flexibility and mental reserve. However, the issue arises when the anxiety becomes a constant. The mind is swept into the constant turbulence of negativity, with no hope in the distance, or the sky from a window.

If this pattern is consistent all through your life span, the likelihood of suffering from cognitive issues increases. In addition, this reality along with other aspects increase the likelihood of suffering from Alzheimer's disease.

The cognitive debt Hypothesis

Robert Howard is a Professor of Psychology within University College London. In the year 2015, as a result of a research study that he conducted, he proposed a widely accepted and well-known concept known as"the cognitive debt theory. According to this theory that repetitive and persistent negative thinking causes damage to the brain , and consequently cognitive declines (debts) as we reach certain levels of age.

Another study conducted to prove this concept, which come to light just a few weeks recently. The researcher Dr. Natalie Marchant from this same university tracked 292 people aged over five years to test this hypothesis.

The information is published within the Journal Alzheimer's & Dementia. They read:

The negative thought pattern and the decline in cognitive function are closely linked. People with a ruminant obsessive and negative thinking pattern may experience difficulties with language, attention, memory and spatial awareness.

Also, a less significant issue is: Magnetic resonances revealed increased amount of tau and beta-amyloid protein that create the standard plaques in neuronsthat block communications between the two. This is a sign of that Alzheimer's disease marker.

The relationship between depression and anxiety in later life

We have learned that cognitive decline and negative thinking decline are closely linked. But, there's an underlying cause. This pattern of reasoning that is devoid of optimism and flexibility, as well as hope and imagination is a result of disorders like depression or anxiety.

This is the information Professor Dr. Amy Gimson points out through her research in the University of Southampton, United Kingdom.

Loneliness and mood disorders

Based on this research it's very frequent for those between 55 and 60 to be suffering from these disorders of the mind that are often linked to family, work, and existential issues. The other reason we notice all too often is the feeling of loneliness.

We are creating a more connected, yet lonely society. We're lacking high-quality connections. We are lacking mechanisms for integrating individuals of all ages into the daily routine in order to make them more social and set goals for the horizon, keep creating connections and cultivating expectations and fantasies towards the future.

All of these elements act as a defense mechanism against cognitive and dementia-related issues. It is not enough to stop Alzheimer's progression, but maybe, we can delay the appearance of Alzheimer's disease and improve longevity and quality of life.

A vicious cycle of anger When emotions trap you

The cycle of anger forms the root of many self-destructive behaviours that can break relationships and trigger unpleasant situations that cause regret in the end. The psychological impact of this aspect can be devastating when we don't control it effectively. The problem is that there are a few of us who are trained in this crucial life-long skill.

Dante set the sins that are committed by anger within his seventh circle. Then, he broke it down into 3 smaller ones and constructed of stone , because according to him, this part of human nature causes us to engage in multiple actions including insults or other types of violence. This hell-zone was guarded by a mythological and powerful character: the minotaur.

There are few emotions that have more negative or negative associations than anger. It is nevertheless important to recognize that anger fulfills its role as a mental point perspective. It is essential in our behavioral and emotional repertoire because anger triggers us to react at injustices, or to something that can hurt us or threatens our moral beliefs.

We all have the right to feel angry However, we need to be aware of how to deal with it. If we handle it with a sense of deliberation we can make the necessary changes that help us regain our equilibrium and feel more comfortable.

It's safe to affirm that anger shares many similarities with fear. In a psychological sense both emotions cause us to avoid certain things or fight against particular thing. There is no any middle ground. The mind and the body is in survival mode since there is something that irritates us, which harms us, and is threatening our integrity in any way. As a result we are compelled to get out or take action.

But, not many people are aware of this feeling. People tend to view anger in a negative way, without realizing that it has a transformative power. It motivates us to act and, generally speaking the act of acting can be an opportunity for change.

Anger that is directed properly can help us to resolve complex problems and issues. However, before doing this we must understand how they work and also the spiral of anger.

What is the reason we feel anger?

Anger is a feeling that may range from anger to rage. It may be triggered by anger, disappointment or even an insult and even injustice, that violates our beliefs and integrity. The same way, the emotion passes through an intense physical reaction identical to anxiety: the heart beats and the muscles become tense and, perhaps most alarmingly the brain is unable to think in a rational manner to allow itself to be controlled by emotion.

Here's a key information about anger that we should be aware of. The emotion can grow in intensity in the event that it is allowed to "feed" it. We are away from being able to manage it. We allow it to grow in strength.

How do we foster or help make this feeling more intense? Through the circle of anger.

Anger is a vicious loop. What is it?

The cycle of anger can be an unwitting trap we build and reinforce through our thoughts. Research like those conducted in researchers from the Texas Department of Psychobiology affect the way this process is activated when anger is extremely extreme.

At that point that the emotion is an emotional dulling. We shut down our ability to reflect and a variety of highly problematic processes start. These are:

* On one side, the trigger is what causes us to feel anger, annoyance or outrage.

* Physiological dimensions. Psychophysiological activation can be extremely intense. It is stressful, impedes us, and puts us in a highly complicated state that we could be screamed at, hit or crying.

* The accumulation of our emotions. In spite of our bodily reactions anger is a tendency to grow; it is absorbed into us, affecting our balanceand distorted the whole.

* Unchanged thoughts. When we suck in our emotions and fail to control them, our

thinking becomes altered and shifts. It's when everything is a problem. When we begin to lose faith, fear anger, frustration and fatigue appear.

* Distorted reality. If thoughts are suspended in anger, negativity and a sense of discontent, the outside world is transformed, everything goes grey, and nothing entices us, or at least we have no interest in anything or anything that causes us to be feel angry. In a matter of seconds we feel an anger and rage that is uncontrollable.

People who are addicted to negativity Six Signs of a Negativity-Affected Person

We all know someone who is prone to view things from an optimistic view. We don't know why however, every time we're around the person, we notice how much worse our mood is and our desire to flee increases by the minute. It's because we've came across one of those individuals who are obsessed with negativity.

They do not seem to take them realize that they are doing a inflicting harm on the people who are around them. Their negativity is infectious and causes others to shun them in the end. They're usually not bad individuals, but they can be extremely difficult in their ways of looking at things. Everyone hates being reminded of all the world's negative aspects.

People who are addicted to negativity can't see the bright side of the hurricane clouds or notice the one cloud that is that is dominated by a sun burning.

If they do not do their part in changing their mindset, we are able to assist them in doing nothing. Therefore, if we are looking to be supportive of them the first thing we have to do is motivate them to take a step in the right direction, and then make the choice.

Six signs that indicate people who are addicted to negative thoughts

1. They fret about insignificant problems

People who are obsessed with negative thoughts drown in the water of a glass. They believe that the breaking of a plate is a global drama that they could swap out for a fresh one in only a couple of hours. They begin to think smugly about the future rather than taking in the present which makes them more negative.

They aren't able to properly assess the importance of every object, or their tendencies to exaggerate a situation can cause the accuser to claim that they are not being reliable. We all remember the tale that was Peter as well as the Wolf and its tragic conclusion.

2. They overlook the positive

It doesn't matter whether they had a good day at work, if they received a present or heard positive news. They are only focused on the aspects of their lives that they do not enjoy, disregarding the positive moments.

They're not aware of their lives by not focusing on positive aspects, and when they think about it, they seem to reach the rational conclusion that they're very poor or that their worth is low. They aren't concerned about their own happiness. They simply remain in the tangle of bad luck that their brain manipulates.

3. They are not able to accept a compliment.

They are not happy when they receive praise or threatens them. The negative feedback also impacts their self-esteem. Any compliment or praise is considered an offence.

They think that other people think they are ridiculing them because they are just trying to please. They are unable to accept that they too are worthy, no matter how difficult it is to believe it.

4. They are only talking about their issues: there is no any room for the problems of the other

They like to display how awful their lives are for them, yet they aren't concerned about how others think. They don't know how to listen and are self-centered Their opinions are always the worst. The handful of times they allow people join in their monologues are due to the fact that they have something they object to. Sometimes, this lack empathy can lead to conflicts with others, particularly when the limits are exceeded.

Naturally, people feel the urge to keep venting and this can be quite stressful.

5. They are very cautious about taking risks.

They fret a lot about what other people think of their opinions of them. Every negative comment is having an unsettling effect on them. They base their opinions on the opinions of others without any objectivity that makes them highly dependent and insecure.

They are so terrified of suffering due to the things that others be saying or doing that they are not afraid to create the corresponding "mental videos" where they are frequently victimized or hurt (something is something we all do and do, enhanced with "special results"). They would rather try a few times by doing this and defend themselves (they believe they have already taken a lot of chances, or that they are on "too many open doors").

6. They may become extremely paranoid.

People who are obsessed with the negative tend to be extremely paranoid. An out of the ordinary laugh or a smile that is a little tense makes them believe that we're speaking ill of them. The result is that people around them become extremely cautious of them, and increases their desire to move off of them.

These actions are difficult to take in and may even be unpalatable. Be cautious and attempt to comprehend why they're doing this.

Most of the time, their actions are the result of an assortment of negative events that were not taken care of properly. It's never too late to re-learn that not everything is white or black We live in grey environment. Bad days and good days will have their places, however not everything is going to be a disaster.

"The Science of Guilt

Guilt is regarded as to be one of those "negative" feelings that we will be faced with in our lives on a variety of occasions. It is not a pleasant emotion because it makes us feel uneasy however, it is essential to change our surroundings.

The emotion is triggered by the perception or feeling of being in violation of social or personal ethical rules towards other people (for whom another person has been injured) or oneself. It is possible to feel a sense of guilt due to the cause, because we have done something we believed we shouldn't have done, or , conversely we didn't do something we believed was right, and we now feel guilty.

Guilt is a process in that, in response to the act or omission of another, we form an "moral decision" of our actions (including your thoughts) and a "rule" that we've committed a wrong, and should be punished. As a judgement we make of our behavior (and our thoughts) guilt is a subjective emotion because it is a part of the judgment we make about our actions. This is why it can be very destructive. Most of the time there isn't a single external fact that triggers the individual's desire to feel guilt for the events that have occurred or been resolved.

Principal aspects of guilt

There are three major components of guilt:

* The cause whether it is real or imagined.

* The negative experience or self-assessment of the action by the individual (bad conscience)

* The unpleasant emotion that comes from guilt (remorse)

Feelings of guilt can lead to feelings of shame, sadness and self-pity. It can trigger an array of emotions which make us feel bad and feed off one another and make it hard to recognize and overcome.

Guilt can be viewed either way:

* Intrinsic: It's the discomfort that comes over us when we commit the act (or the lack from

it) and has been hurt as a result. For instance passing an exam and failing , and then contemplating, "If I had studied more ..." I would have felt ashamed for not having prepared enough to be able to take the test and get it passed.

External: The issue occurs when we perform the behavior (or its absence) which means that someone else (different from us) is hurt. For instance, you're involved in an argument with a person and you are disrespectful to him causes your friend to feel wounded. It makes you feel guilty for having caused harm to the person.

How can guilt manifest itself?

Sometimes, the sense of guilt may become so intense that it will clearly manifest itself in the following indicators:

• Physical: Psychophysiological manifestation of of guilt manifests as discomfort in the stomach, chest and head. It can also be felt in the pressure of the head and back, as well as pain in your back.

* Emotional: Irritability, anxiety and, often we refer to it as a feeling similar to sadness.

* Cognitive Self-reproaches and self-accusations and negative thoughts about self-esteem and self-worth.

When guilt becomes to pathological

An emotion can become pathological if it is experienced repeatedly, usually over time, it can become an extremely strong and intrusive emotion, to the point that it affects our daily routine. We cease to function on different levels (work or social, as well as family) and then we fall to the mercy of our emotions.

Guilt can become pathological through excessive guilt, and in the process there is a denial of awareness in both situations. The overt or inexplicably strong feeling of guilt is connected to depression, and is one of the symptoms of depressive episodes that cause the sufferer to continually self-recriminate. It is normal to feel guilty over being depressed as well as not being able think the way that others do.

The presence of guilt-related pathology is also evident in the obsessive-compulsive disorder (characterized by its high demands and obsession with perfection) also in phobias as well as addictions. In such instances guilt plays a role as a part of the issue. It's not healthy guilt that can cause a change or alter behaviour. Instead, it functions as an element of continuous emotional punishment that generally increases the severity of the problem.

The feelings of guilt and shame are extremely intense, and are stemming from minor incidents or minor guilt from the past that now become an unfathomable mountain of unworthiness and harm. Examples: "I am a monster," "I am worth nothing," "I am to blame for the demise of ...". This means that the person feels guilty despite not having committed an act of omission or perhaps not knowing the reason.

This type of guilt that is based on actions beyond the control of a person, is harmful and stops them from experiencing satisfaction from the actions they carry out properly. Since they go unnoticed their value and significance. Ultimately, it is about enjoying living a full and fulfilling life.

There are many kinds and types of negativity that could hurt your health. These are typically automatic thoughts Some of them are simply thoughts that have been repressed; which is, the thoughts that parents and other important adults imparted to you during your early years and that you carry throughout your life. Others negative thoughts arise as a result of a flawed perspective of life or not meeting expectations.

Albert Ellis, the creator of the rational and emotional behavior therapy, was convinced that what is important to us isn't the way we experience it, however, it is our interpretation. The interpretations we make take form as negative thoughts that cause discomfort, and even more they hinder our from finding a satisfying solution to our problems , since they tend to perpetuate a cycle of negative thoughts. The first step in breaking out of the loop is to be aware of all kinds and types of negativity that may be a constant source of anxiety.

Are you a victim these kinds of thoughts that are negative?

The number of kinds of negativity as the people however, they can be categorized into eight major categories that are easy to identify through the attitude they create.

1. A permanent emergency state

When you experience something, you view it as an emergency. This is due to the fact that your amygdala gets activated and you are able to only hear the alarm message. An emotional hijacking takes place in your brain, creating the panic response. If you imagine that it is an emergency, you respond in a way that is not normal. This kind of a catastrophic mindset can cause you to overestimate the risks and underestimate your capabilities to tackle difficulties. This type of thinking can be extremely risky as it creates an attitude of helplessness that has been learned.

2. Self-saboteur

If you face any difficulty and you instantly sabotage yourself. You take every incident in your own hands and think you are responsible for events that you cannot control. Your negative thoughts block you from thinking rationally so you reprimand and blame yourself on a regular basis. This means that every whenever a problem happens you feel depressed and lose confidence in yourself. This a way of thinking that makes you the person you are most at risk as you'll always fall.

3. The extreme

If an event occurs, you only discern the extremes. This kind of thinking, sometimes referred to as dichotomous makes you view the world as the black-and-white spectrum, and all or nothing, with no middle ground. It is difficult to come up with the right solution without thinking about the variety of grays and other colors. You'll experience an overwhelming amount of stress since you believe that every decision will be a point of no return.

4. The tagger

Whatever happens, we categorize the situation in negative terms since you are only able to be aware of the dramatic effects that the situation could have. The issue is that when applying these labels you are unable to imagine the possibilities the situation could have and you block the way to resolving the issue. This kind of negative thinking could also lead you to define yourself, and eventually create a the impression of yourself and the possibilities you have.

5. Tunnel vision

If you are facing an issue you will notice that your vision instantly diminished, similar to when you walk into an underground tunnel. It is only possible to focus on the negative aspects that are problems, mistakes and flaws. You are unable to see positive aspects, opportunities or strengths, and you are swept into the downward spiral of negativity. This kind of negative thinking is based upon the phenomenon of selective attention. In reality, it's like wearing sunglasses and blinders so that you could only be able to see a small portion of the world, and ignoring the most important aspect in order to solve.

6. The generalizer

If you are faced with a problem the mind starts to wander and you begin to create loose connections between your current and previous things. These connections can lead you to make incorrect and negative generalizations. They are recognized by the way words such as "never," "always," or "all" are frequently used. This kind of generalization typically can lead to what's commonly referred to as the "fortune teller's error" which is the act of jumping into conclusions regarding something that hasn't actually happened but, assuming that the consequences or results could be catastrophic. Naturally, with every assertion, you'll lose some self-esteem and self-confidence, and you are resigned to a negative cycle.

7. The fake

You are constantly focusing on the positives you see in others while minimizing your own strengths and talents due to the fact that you're prone to comparing yourself to others. This negative mindset makes you feel as if you're an unworthy person, and that you do not deserve the things you're able to achieve. You're afraid that people might discover that you're not very smart, skilled and kind and the result is that you've got an issue with your self-esteem. It is common to be affected by what's commonly referred to as "mind-reading," a phenomenon that is where you assume what other people are thinking.

8. The superhero

You wear your cape laid out You strive to never let anyone down. You are proud of doing regardless of what it takes. Your life is dictated with "must" as well as "should" until the point where you completely do not know what you would like to achieve. The issue is that every when you realize that you're not able to help the planet, the self-confidence decreases and you are afflicted with extreme discontent. This is among the most destructive types of negative thoughts since you see things about "duties" as well as "obligations," allowing your life, your choices and your state of mind to completely depend on the actions of others.

The "Two" sides of Doubting

Doubting is okay. It lets us think about our thoughts. It forces us to reflect on our experiences. It aids us in making choices, and to consider our desires or the actions we've accomplished. Our doubts reflect our prudence , and sometimes of our smugness to not take anything for granted.

The best of certain people is always in be in doubt. They admire those who take everything taken for granted, and are regarded as very secure individuals. Doubting is good even if we get off-guard and we like to be apprehensive about certainties. What's what is the distinction between regular doubts and obsessional ones?

Are doubts always "healthy"?

It appears that this isn't the situation. This is confirmed by a variety of problems that sufferers suffering from anxiety disorders where uncertainty has been the mainstay of their lives. And instead of helping them overcome the mysteries that they may have they are engulfed in a trance-like state that they believe they are unable to leave.

What differentiates obsessive doubts from the normal doubts we all face at times?

Differentialities between normal doubts and obsessive doubts

* Common doubts arise with clear evidence of the five senses in the right context.

Common doubts are solved rapidly once the required information is gathered.

Normal doubts are gone when the person is convinced that they've accomplished what's essential from a logic standpoint by making use of common sense.

* Obsessive doubts block the evidence at the time they are beyond the senses.

* The number of obsessive thoughts increases as you consider them.

* In obsessive questions, the person is never sure what he's trying to find. It's always an ambiguous "maybe."

Let's look at some examples of common questions: "What will I eat in the morning?" This normal doubt is supported by specific evidence or facts and is conducted in a manner that is appropriate. Maybe the person is unsure of what she'll eat the next day because she would like to have her food prepared or already cooked. Maybe tomorrow you'll not have the time to think of a new recipe and knowing ahead of time the dishes to cook will help you save time the following day.

The doubts can be easily answered once the correct details are gathered for it. In the case of the above example this happened when the person was mentally planning the menu that he will eat on the next day. When doing this from a rational perspective the person is aware that all he can accomplish to answer the question is accomplished. Doubt mentally create the menu, and then the uncertainty is over.

What about obsessive questions? For instance: "Will I have terminal cancer?" (In a hypochondriacal image). The question arises without evidence or in a wrong context. The individual will go, for instance regularly to the doctor without being able to prove of any health issue and will continue to test their body, without any evidence to support the decision.

Even when logic and common sense inform you that you don't have indication of an illness that is serious The desire to investigate is stronger and the suspicion will rise with the amount of tests or reviews.

By looking at these instances We can determine if the question is normal or when the question is pathological. If people are engrossed in, as we have mentioned previously in persistent doubts which aren't justified by the environment that they are in it is essential to intervene psychologically.

The aim is to help individuals to differentiate between their regular and obsessive doubts to enable them to accept the uncertainty to which we all have to expose ourselves, and be able to discern the aspects of their personality that can cause a person to be addicted to an obsessional question that has a variety of themes.

Negative Thoughts the Power They Hold Over Your Life

Negative thoughts, which are part of your inner conversation, and that you experience every day. Sometimes , you are conscious of them, but sometimes (most) of the time, you're in the dark. This article we'll discuss the elements of your behavior based on cognitive psychology, the ways that negative self-talk can lead to psychological problems The most frequent features and types of thoughts that are negative, as well as how to recognize and overcome these thoughts. We'll leave you at end of this article with the document that includes exercises you can attempt to begin to understand your inner dialogue.

In accordance with the Cognitive Current The thoughts are the ones that underlie every psychological problem. Everything you do is comprised of three main elements: THOUGHTS, Emotions, and ACTIONS.

The three components are linked to one another, and each has an impact on each other in such an approach that when you are looking to alter something, you need to concentrate on altering any of three elements to ensure that the other three components "accompany the change."

Everything you do is comprised of three essential elements: Emotions, Thoughts and actions.

The Greek philosopher Epictetus wrote, "It is not what happens to us, but what we think we say about ourselves." This is what we be said. You should be aware that you are not seeing the world as it is, instead you see the world from the perspective of your mind map. perception and perspective.

Based on what your inner conversation is going, this is the way in which you see the world. If you view the world in a cloak of negative thoughts, such as, "I'm worthless," "I'm extremely bad at this, "life is unfair, " "I'm unfortunate," nothing ever comes out in the right way," ... you'll begin to create negative feelings that go along with the thoughts, and most of all, you'll pretend that you have very bad luck, or weren't worth anything or that the world was hostile.

Based on the law of self-fulfilling prophecy, which describes Cognitive Psychology: if you believe something, feel it and then act accordingly and then, eventually the reality will exactly as you imagined it , because you created it. Imagine that you think your partner isn't trustworthy and is likely to break up with you.

If you begin to feel guilty or angry. you'll start treating your partner in a way that is sour, and behave as if certain that they were not faithful ... the situation becomes very stressful. is extremely difficult for your partner and ultimately, they will leave you. It is likely that your partner has never been infidelity to you, and so your snarky behavior was not logical but at the end of the day you will get what you've always feared most.

The majority of the time we don't realize the influence to our own thoughts. the harm they can bring about and how they can affect our lives. Only those who have managed to break out of the negative circle and begin to think positively and act in that manner have been capable of seeing what happens when whenever you are looking for something positive it is all about getting to get it.

In this case, you could begin to consider "I'm worthy of it," "I merit a promotion," and that will create a positive feeling and self-confidence, which will make you more probable that you'll speak to your boss, request the promotion, and that you will get it from him. you. I'm not going to frighten you. I'm not claiming that if you discuss your situation with your boss you'll get promoted However, I am sure you will have a higher likelihood of receiving it than if believe that you're not worthy of and that you'll not be able to succeed at your job.

Why it is so difficult to alter our internal conversation?

Since virtually all negative thoughts we've had were subconscious. They could be visualizations (mental pictures) and words (with the use of words) that are spontaneously generated. It was psychiatrist Aaron T. Beck was the first person to formulate the most important theory-based framework for addressing these issues in his research and concludes that they were the most direct to depression-related factors.

He also stated that they are extremely difficult to change since they are an internal conversation. We accept them as real and valid without any questionnaires. They are a an integral part of us. It has been confirmed to be the main directly responsible for anxiety issues and obsessive compulsive disorders.

Positive Thoughts: Characteristics

They're uninvoluntary, non-conscious They are not your choice whether or not you will experience them however, they appear spontaneously whenever something happens to you in the course of the daytime. They are not controlled prior to when they manifest. We are only able to act upon their appearance.

They also have a pessimistic element that describes your life in a shocking, devastating tragic, and sad manner ...

They are superficial and distorted and do not perceive reality objectively or in a rational way, and draw conclusions from a small amount of data.

The basis of these are the needs and demands that create a emotionally charged charge on them " I have to be able to pass the test or else I'll be a failure "I need to find a partner by the date of the end of the year or else I'll be on my own "

These are specific: When we start to feel down or anxious, it is typically an extremely specific reason to blame it on, and which we repeatedly think for ourselves ... Are there thoughts you think about throughout the day? ... " He will quit for me, "they will terminate my boss "I have a disease, but I'm not going to recover, "I have no money " ...

They are repetitive: Human living beings are thought to can think about 60,000 times a each day. Recurring thoughts comprise the largest percent of those thoughts. What do you think about the most?

They are reliable They are not backed by any convincing evidence to support their claims, but you trust they are true. It is "absolute factual statements."

A test you could use is to share these thoughts, or to try to observe them objectively. Most likely, the person you are talking to won't see it as very well, or from afar and you think it's "ridiculous."

Chapter 3: The Negativity Bias

Cognitive biases are psychological phenomena which alter our perception of the information recorded by our senses, leading to confusion, distortion, or incorrect interpretation of the data we've got.

Social prejudices can be applied to prejudices in the way we identify and disrupt our relationships in our daily lives with others.

Cognitive Biases: How the Mind deceives us

As a natural necessity the phenomenon of cognitive biases evolved to allow humans to take immediate decisions, which the brain makes to respond rapidly to certain situations, stimuli or conditions, that could be difficult to comprehend all information due to their complexity. They require specific or subjective filtering.

Cognitive bias may cause us to make mistakes. It allows us to make decisions quicker or to make an emotional judgement in situations where the immediate nature of the situation doesn't allow for logical examination.

Cognitive Psychology studies this kind of phenomena as well as other techniques and structures that are used to process information.

Prejudice concept or cognitive bias

Prejudice or cognitive bias is a result from various processes that aren't readily discernible. They include heuristic processes (mental shortcuts) moral and emotional motives, as well as social influences.

It was the idea of cognitive bias that was first introduced through Daniel Kahneman in 1972, after he realized that people were unable to make sense of huge amounts. Kahneman as well as other scientists discovered the existence of scenarios patterns that showed that the decisions and judgments weren't dependent on predictability as per the theory of rational choice.

They explained these variations by locating the cause of heurism. intuition-based processes which are often the cause of systematic errors.

The research on cognitive biases expanded their scope, and different disciplines were also examining these biases, including the fields of medicine and political sciences. The result was the development of the discipline of Behavioral Economics. It was elevated to the status of Kahneman when he won the Nobel Prize in Economics in 2002, for integrating the study of psychology into economic science by identifying connections between the human mind and in the process of making decisions.

But, certain people who are critical of Kahneman assert that heuristics must not cause us to think of human thinking as a jumble of cognitive biases that are irrational and inclinations, but rather to see rationality as a tool for adaptive use that doesn't blend with the formal logic rules or probabilistic.

The most known cognitive biases are studied.

* Retrospective bias, also known as A posteriori bias: It's the habit of interpreting the past as predictable events.

* Correspondence bias or errors when attribution is made: This is a tendency to exaggerate the rationales of other people's actions or personal experience.

* Confirmation bias: It's the tendency to reinforce beliefs about how to discover or make sense of information.

* Self-service bias The desire to assume more accountability for failure than success. When we tend to think of the lack of knowledge as a good thing for the purpose and it's also demonstrated.

False consensus bias: It's the tendency to conclude that, in the presence of others, your beliefs and opinions, values and customs are more widespread than they actually are.

"Memory bias": the meaning of our memories can be distorted through memory bias.

A bias in representation when we think that something is more likely to happen from an assumption that does not provide a prediction for something.

A good example to show cognitive biases: Bouba or Kiki

The bouba/kiki effect is among of the most widely known cognitive biases. It was first discovered in 1929 by Estonian scientist Wolfgang Kohler. In an experiment conducted in Tenerife (Spain) the scientist showed various shapes to participants. They observed a strong preference from the subjects who associated the pointed shape to the term "takete" while the rounded form by the name "baluba."

It was 2001 when V. Ramachandran conducted the same experiment by using the terms "kiki" as well as "bouba," and many people were asked which one of the forms was known as "bouba" as well as which was referred to as "kiki."

Over 90% of people voted for the round shape to be "bouba" while the pointed form was referred to "kiki." This gave an experiment to understand that the human brain can extract features in abstract sound and shapes.

Recent research conducted by Daphne Maurer showed that even youngsters under the age of three (who aren't yet reading) already experience this effect.

The Kiki/Bouba effect: explanations

Ramachandran and Hubbard consider the kiki/bouba effect as a proof of the implications for the development of human language, since it provides clues that the way in which we name certain objects isn't entirely random.

A call to the rounded form "bouba" may indicate that this bias comes from the manner in which we say the word by placing the mouth being in a more rounded position to produce the sound, and we make use of an angular and more tense sound that resembles the "kiki" sounds.

It is important to note it is important to note that sounds in the letters "k" are more harsh than the sounds in "b." The presence of this kind of "synesthetic maps" suggests that this type of phenomenon could be the basis for auditory symbolism where phonemes are mapped and linked to particular objects and things in a non-arbitrary fashion.

Autism sufferers, however don't show an overwhelming preference. The subjects who were examined scored over 90% when they attribute "bouba" due to its rounded shape , and "kiki" due to its angle, the proportion falls to 60% in individuals with autism.

The Halo Effect

The"halo effect" ("halo impact" is a term used in English) is a form of prejudice or cognitive bias resulting from the tendency to assess positively certain aspects of a person based on the perception that one holds about him: Human beings tend to generalize based on one characteristic.

Imagine, for instance, you have a friend you admire and you be inclined to define it using traits that have positive aspects even if we don't have any relevant details regarding the person. The Halo effect is present every day and in a variety of situations.

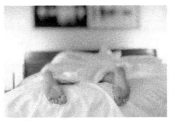

The Halo Effect, one certain aspect is highlighted as dominant or that is distinct from the beginning. This feature can cause us to attribute a distortion to it. It is interesting with any kind of quality, if it is relevant to the person who will be evaluating them.

It's an effect that is mysterious that acts as an element that prompts us to think deeply when working on behalf of a brand, and think about the market segment it is targeting.

The definition of the term refers to Edward L. Thorndike, an American psychologist and pedagogue who was who was a precursor of behavioral psychology. In the early 1920s, while conducting one of his army studies he noticed that when evaluating the officers for the soldiers there was a significant correlation between the positive and negative characteristics This means that when you look at you look at the different characteristics of an individual are assessed, either the either the most positive or negative are revealed.

The combination of both is not typically offered, even though it is logical. In his research, Thorndike found a high correlation between attractiveness to the physical, intelligence and character. This is which later research studies confirm. A person with a good appearance is often perceived to be thoughtful and generous. Physical attractiveness is one the most influential factors in the"halo effect.

The effect could have catastrophic consequences and can sour opportunities can hinder or hinder those who are around us We are in a world full of looks in which beauty is a way to be seen which makes it much easier for many to attain goals and to be valued as an attribute that is positive to his appearance, with a flawless smile, and a manner of dressing. However, those who do not conform to this model, he will be instantly rejected for numerous factors, including the prospect of finding a partner.

Making judgments about value is that is normal to humans and we perform it with no malice. The reason for this is that it's evolutionary because it is through this process that we can anticipate the possibility of aggression. These perceptions are generally due to social learning (family friends, media, friends, etc.) and, through them, we'll be conditioned in our relationships.

A number of studies have shown that within 7 seconds we can form an opinion about the things we see. The value judgment we form determines our expectations and also our manner of communicating with that person.

According to Social psychologist Solomon Asch, physical attractiveness is the most desirable quality that is the basis of the"halo" effect. Physical attractiveness is one of the variables which most strongly evokes the effect of the halo. Physical attractiveness offers people tangible details about the effect of halo, and it's certain aspects of physical attractiveness that are most effective in triggering the halo effect.

These particular traits help us evaluate the personality of an individual. There are many of these traits are specific to a person (for instance hair color, eye color and weight).

For instance anyone who is considered attractive because of a portion of their physical appearance are also thought of as intelligent or generous. Numerous studies have confirmed the importance of attractiveness in creating the"halo effect.

A new study found that attractiveness can influence our perceptions of the person's life, achievements and character. The study found that attractiveness was associated with weight. People who were perceived to be attractive were rated as more pleasant as well as more trustworthy. However, Harol Kelly's, in his theory of personality states that the impression that we get from someone will impact how we perceive the person in the future. We can also identify traits like being warm emotional, supportive and sincere, loving and professional.

In the realm of marketing, this effect is an interesting idea to think about. It's a kind of cognitive bias that occurs when one's impression of certain quality is influenced by perception of the traits that have occurred before in a series of possible interpretations. For instance, when a brand chooses to adopt an elite athlete, actor, singer, or other kind of famous persona. The brand automatically achieves the Halo effect that comes with the celebrity's favorable image standing, and the public perceives the perception of the celebrity based on that.

If you also have an opinion on an item from a specific brand, you'll be prone to have a similar impression of other products from that same manufacturer, even though you don't have any objective evidence to support your decision. Companies make use of the Halo effect to their advantage. by employing different strategies to broaden positive perceptions of their brand, and to minimize negative reviews. This article will show you how businesses do to leave an impression that is positive:

1. Create a product that is not competing The most effective method of standing out in the marketplace will be to first come up with something. Apple did this by releasing the cult iPod. It was so well-received it Apple computers also saw sales increase. This is an obvious halo effect. When the iPod is great, then the computers from the same model must be equally good.

2. Make sure you link your image with that of a celebrity You've surely seen a variety of examples on TV and on posters. For instance, footballers often appear in ads. Football is the world's most well-known sportand we all know that footballers earn a lot of dollars. Therefore, any brand with there is a soccer player sends out messages that convey glamour and class.

In the classrooms of compulsory education there is also the halo effect to be more desirable. It's evident in the well-known "labels" which teachers give their students. It's a thing that happens often without intention due to the fact that we all are familiar with assessing the world within us.

If you've figured out that your student is brilliant They will eventually feel that they are more valuable. So, they'll try more hard and, in the absence of conscious thought the teacher may allow the student to get some good results , without the student noticing.

It is also the case when evaluating. When you're evaluating an open-ended test it is understood that the score that is given to the initial question is the basis for how the rest will be judged. Teachers must know this fact and behave with the absolute manner that is possible.

Halo effect on Human Resources

This is also the case also in Human Resources, specifically in two areas: selection of personnel and evaluations of performance.

The halo effect is a common feature of an interview for personnel selection falling into the web that cause this phenomenon is among the most frequently made mistakes in interviews for selection, and it's because the first characteristics we observe on others affect the way we perceive it during the interview process. One aspect that can be the most influential factor in the effect is the attractiveness of people as we mentioned in the previous paragraph. Someone who is considered to be attractive or beautiful is typically more valued, even though they possess fewer capabilities or skills than someone with no physical beauty. However, it has been established that physical appearance is not the only factor which can cause prejudices, which can lead that it gives the opportunity to certain individuals over others. It is also important to think about the effect of halo in selection because of social networks. They are now an additional factor in judging to select the best candidate for the job as well as your curriculum vitae. There are studies that show that over 60% of employers utilize more than two different social networking sites for meeting potential candidates.

The halo effect is a part of evaluation of performance: They can be used to assess the effectiveness of resources to meet the objectives in the various areas of the organization. The process of evaluating performance is based on regular checks wherein deficiencies in the efficiency of resources are identified. In the course of performance evaluations managers may make a mistake about the subject. The halo effect could occur due to an assessment solely based on one aspect like the appearance of the person or their behavior. Recent behavior is the determining factor of the evaluation regardless of how an employee has been doing over the course of time. In this instance the supervisor could highly review an employee who performed well during the past week, and disregard his previous actions. A typical situation of an adverse halo effect is the existence of prejudices in the workplace when a manager is inclined to judge the performance of a worker more negatively because of their race, gender or religion.

Halo effect as well as Devil effect

The halo effect and Satan effect comprise two aspects of the one coin. These cognitive biases can be traced to their roots in our brain's tendency to simplify things and drawing conclusions from inertia instead of performing the analysis of each detail in isolation.

"The devil" ("devil effects" to use English) (also known as the reverse halo effect), is identical with the same halo effects however in reverse. It occurs when particular features of a person are judged negative when the overall perception of the person is negative.

In the case of the devil effect we will use the historical figure Mao Tse-Tung. Many people criticize Mao for having instituted the totalitarian system in China. However, not many will applaud the social and economic successes it made in their country (for instance, it was able to make the majority of China educated, increasing from 15 percent in 1949, to 80percent in the year 1970. It also transformed the country that was poor into a world-class power) due to the bad image we see to deal with in the West.

However, how can we stay clear of the effects of devil and halo? Like other cognitive prejudices they aren't impossible to get rid of The best method to determine the quality of someone is to ask yourself: would we be thinking exactly the same way about this particular aspect if we were somebody else?

In the world of politics, if you consider a person who is a part of a style as attractive, then most people would think that their method of conducting politics also has attractive aspects which are extremely positive for the person. It is possible that, in the campaigning for elections, just before an election, some of the candidates attempt to show empathy, closeness and compassion.

A few examples of the Halo Effect, and the devil effect.

There are many instances that show the effect of halo as well as the effect of devil. In the world of marketing the halo effect generally is experienced by consumers who purchased a particular product and were happy with the outcome which leads them to view the other products in a very positive manner. This is among the main reasons Apple has gained customer loyalties to its products.

For the illustration of the devil's effect, I'll use an article published in The Guardian, an English paper "The Guardian" which examines the devil effect of Hugo Chavez. The devil effect causes few people appreciate Venezuela's accomplishments in terms of education and health because of the negative image that was portrayed within and around the West of the persona of the president of Venezuela, Hugo Chavez.

*Warning: By presenting this scenario I am not trying to support a corrupt, economically deficient government, like that of the Venezuelan one. I am only trying to provide an extreme case of this cognitive bias.

The Negativity Bias

The Negativity Bias is a psychological condition that makes people tend to pay more attention and give more importance to negative experiences over positive ones. Positive stimuli are more visible and dominant, while responses to negative and unpleasant events are stronger and faster than those that respond to opportunities or pleasures.

Poor parents, bad emotions and poor feedback are more damaging than positive ones, and negative information gets processed prior to positive information. This is a phenomenon that is so widespread and spans a variety of human experience areas that it is the fundamental rule of psychology. We will be able to see instances of this bias in various fields and, at the end, we will discover the evolutionary explanation for the phenomenon. I will present the principal conclusions of the research without giving the full details of them;

The psychology books dedicate more chapters than uncomfortable emotions than they do to pleasant ones. In a study of 17,000 psychology journal articles 69% focused on negative issues while 31% were devoted to positive issues.

There are more terms for negative emotions than positive ones. Averill created an atlas of 558 words used to describe emotions, and found 62% negative words and 38 percent positive. It appears that it's more important to define and talk about bad emotions than to discuss positive ones. It is also more difficult and employ more methods to avoid negative emotions rather than to create positive ones. They also remember bad emotions with increasing time and effort is spent working through them.

It is important for people to know the reasons behind what happens to them and research suggests the idea that people think deeper and try to understand the meaning of the events that occur to us. When things that are good occur for us, we do not usually think about why it happens to us. We just go on with our lives. The threat of aggressive characters are better spotted in different tests than neutral or nice faces. In the world of journalism, it's widely known that good news isn't news.

The media is often called upon to share the good news, but these efforts usually fail. Similar happens in the world of the realm of literature. Fiedler reviewed the development of novels and stated that nobody had been able to write a book about the joys of a happily marriage however, marital conflicts are present in many novels.

In the area of human relationships there are many instances. In a variety of studies on couples who are married, Gottman finds that negative affects are reciprocated more frequently in comparison to positive effects, reducing satisfaction in relationships.

It's not important to do something good in order to compensate, if you've committed a crime. Gottman suggests that positive and beneficial interactions must outweigh negative in five to 1. If the ratio is lower then the marriage is at risk. good chance of falling apart.

This implies that the long-term viability of a business depends more on doing good things rather instead of doing positive things. Similar thing occurs with regard to sexuality Sexual dysfunction can have more impact on the relationship than a healthy sexual function.

McCarthy observes that when sexuality is positive within the relationship, it is responsible for 15 percent of the couples' variance however, if the relationship is not good or even nonexistent the relationship is accounted for by 50% to 65 percent. Sexual experiences that are not pleasant will therefore outweigh positive ones in the marriage. A study sought to determine which element most affected the development of friendships in residence and discovered the factor was closeness. intimacy in coexistence.

However, as they continued to research the effects of being close to each other increased the chance that two individuals would end up becoming enemies more than the probability that they would eventually become friends as predicted. Because bad events are more likely than good ones, a greater proximity to one another can cause more enemies than friends.

Regarding learning, it's inconvenient to state that, however, even though textbooks state that rewards are better than punishment to learn However, there isn't any solid proof. The books that Baumeister has reviewed show that, in fact, that punishment can be more effective in fostering studying than rewarding.

Concerning aversive conditioning, it can be accomplished rapidly, and sometimes in only one exposure. However the process of conditioning preferences by positive stimuli is typically more gradual. The brain's reaction towards negative stimulus is more powerful at the neuronal level, as demonstrated by Smith's research of the P1-P1 connection, that show higher P1-potentials in response to them than when presented with positive stimuli.

When we think about how we react to situations, we notice that events that are bad have longer-lasting impact and more severe consequences than good events. The impact of positive events is less noticeable. The lottery winners are quick to return, after initial excitement back to their usual level of joy.

However the victims of misfortune require longer for adjustment to situation since they constantly think about the previous state in which is what Brickman described as "The the nostalgia effects." The pain that comes with losing money more than the thrill in winning.

It hurts the more when you lose $50, than the excitement in winning it. The drive to avoid losing something is higher than the desire to be a winner of something.

In the field of sexuality it is evident that a single incident of trauma could result in devastating consequences for the rest of your life. However, there doesn't appear to be a reverse of trauma. It is the "anti-trauma," a single positive sexual experience that brings positive effects equivalent to the damage that is that is caused by an experience that is traumatic to the sexual. A good day or a bad one does affect how the following day will unfold, while an unpleasant day can affect how we will feel the following day.

Morally knowing something that is negative about a person or acquaintance has more weight, far more than having a good impression. Reputations that are bad are easy to get and are difficult to fix, whereas good ones are difficult to obtain and simple to lose. It doesn't matter if ministers visit hospitals every day for 200 days.

If we discover the employee does not pay his social security assistant, he will be permanently discredited and lost. Because good behavior is often and expected, bad behaviour is more evident and crucial to be aware of. To be classified as good, one must always be a good person in order to be categorized as bad, one doesn't necessarily have to be immoral constantly so any immoral act can be interpreted as an indicator (it is fascinating to note that all things happen when you are intelligent an extremely clever act can cause an individual to be regarded as intelligent even though the person later commits a number of foolish things). Take a look.

After a wrong act was committed it's extremely difficult to erase it with positive actions. The initial impression created by moral wrongdoing is difficult to alter. In the course of a study, participants had to be asked about the number of were required to be saved from their own lives a person who killed someone in order to clean his actions (he was required to save them one at a time and put his life at risk).

It was found that he was required to save at least 25 people on average. One study found that the participants could be asked the number of could be saved from their lives in the event that someone killed someone to cover up his crime (had to save them one at a time and put his life at risk).

In the realm of health, we know that stress can lower the immune system. However, relaxation hasn't produced positive results for a capacity comparable to stress ' negative sense. Studies conducted with medical students who were instructed how to relax, they did not increase the immune system.

It's also been observed that social support doesn't increase immunity, however the absence of social support and loneliness can significantly deteriorate it. In a study on cancer patients optimism was not a predictor of survival, while pessimism was able to predict mortality among the young. Another study has demonstrated that pessimism, but not optimism, is a predictor of an optimal course of cancer.

In addition there are studies that show that writing about negative events, such as anxiety, depression and so on. boosts your immunity and overall health. Health is a major factor in our happiness even when it's negative. If it's good it's impact is minimal or even negligible.

Its Negativity Bias and Evolution

Why do we have this Negativity Bias? It is a pattern that is prevalent throughout all domains of our psychological research, which is also observed in animals and children in the early years, makes us to look at theories that don't require any language or cultural background.

While various theories have been suggested but it is inevitable to consider evolutionary theory to discover where this particular characteristic of our brain is derived from: events that are bad have more power than good ones. This is because they are more adaptable, and reacting to the world around us in this way helps to ensure the survival of our species.

Each of Rozin and Baumeister both agree on this both, however Baumeister gives more attention to the evolutionary perspective. Through our evolution organisms that are adjusted to deal with threats have survived and have been capable of passing on their genes.

Someone who doesn't take advantage of an opportunity might regret it later however nothing bad occurred. There are other chances. But, the one who does not take the risk once could be injured or even killed. The survival of the fittest requires urgent and specific attention to events that are dangerous, while handling good events is more awaited.

The negative things also can indicate that we need to change something within us. They force self-regulation. Through self-regulation, an organism adapts itself to its environment. The organism that adheres to the same behaviors that were successful in the past might not be able to tackle the dangers and issues of the modern times.

Examining the issue from an evolutionary angle, we can know why positive actions result in less long-lasting effects as bad actions. If pleasure and satisfaction were eternal, we'd not have the motivation to continue moving forward to gain more rewards.

The temporary nature of positive emotions will result in the development of the human race which is adaptable. If negative feelings were to disappear, people are likely to repeat their mistakes and risk evaporating. A second argument in support of this belief is that good is an unwaveringness in the course of time, and can't be created by one positive event, but could be destroyed by one single incident.

Good events require stability, due to the asymmetry between death and life: an person will live for many years in the event that he can survive every day. There isn't a perfect experience which can counteract the impact of being unlucky for a day. It is not worth taking time and effort seeking out the best experiences, but with the intention of failing to live.

To see what life might be like in a world where the good was more powerful in comparison to the evil, let's take a look at those who suffer from the condition of congenital insensitivity to pain. They feel more comfortable than pain-inducing sensations, however they are often young.

They are afflicted with burns as well as amputations and bone injuries as a result of not being aware of the need to adjust their posture and place their hands on the hot heater, and experience trauma of all sorts. People who are not sensitive towards guilt (psychopaths) are a different category that is rejected by society and lose the benefits the group can provide.

Everything we've that has been discussed thus far suggests that it's logical to assume that we are genetically conditioned to pay more concentration to negative events. Thus, we have a glimpse of the benefits evolution has to offer us with insight into the function of our human brain.

The evolutionary view will allow us to establish the foundations needed for an accurate understanding of them. response"Why? "Why?" This isn't the end of the word, not even close to it but over the top of that foundation there's a ton of taxonomic work to be done and an abundance of research to be done yet we have a foundation to build upon.

Last but not least, I wanted to put a difficult issue which requires my solution. While reading this article the article, you may were thinking that living in the shadows of this bias can make things not always fair at times. What could we do in the interest of building an ideal world, take action to stop some manifestations of this bias?

The reasoning behind the negativity bias

An easy "good" isn't enough to express enthusiasm. It needs to be communicated in a more pronounced manner. A negative assessment however is not in need of any more support. This is known as the negative bias. Recently, Christine Liebrecht of the University of Tilburg and her team have looked into the ways in which this "linguistic injustice" could be addressed.

This study asked companions to read a short text on the exchange between person A and B. They exchanged opinions about their own experience at restaurants. The participants thought that the comment "The food was excellent" was less arousing than the statement "The food was not good."

The same effect was seen in the adjective pairs "smart" as well as "silly," "exciting," and "boring," "pretty," and "ugly." The negative words usually made an impression more strongly over positive words.

When the researchers amplified up the positive adjectives (with words such as "wonderful") and the negative bias decreased. Participants also perceived "very excellent" as being more powerful than "bad." But, if they contrasted the meaning of "very good" to "very poor," the latter carried more importance than the positive one.

The authors aren't too amazed by the findings that, generally speaking, in our interpersonal interactions, we are able to express ourselves positively. The word "good" can be the first step. This is why negative comments seem to have more weight because they are seldom used in a social setting. In addition, negative remarks be a signal that people would not wish to overlook under any circumstance.

The Negativity Bias: How it affects our thinking

How many of us been more concerned about hearing things that aren't true than saying something positive? Humans attach more value to what we perceive as negative than the things we think are positively or even neutral.

It is now clear that the negativity bias or the negativity effect, gives more significance to the negative elements of an particular person, event or circumstance. This is the result of giving more importance to negative events over neutral or positive. This psychological phenomenon has also been called positivity-negativity asymmetry and has a significant impact on our daily lives.

This, for instance, helps us comprehend the reason why people, when they meet someone new and discover the negative traits they have tend to concentrate on their negative traits. This can create an unfavourable first impression which is difficult to alter in the long run.

It is also why people tend to be more aware of moments in which a type of tragic event took place or we have not enjoyed, than those which were pleasant. There are more insults to our minds than praise. we respond in a more intense way to negative events rather than positive ones and we are more likely to think more often, of the negative prior to the good that has occurred to us.

Elements that form the phenomena

In order to explain the negative bias, research team of Paul Rozin and Edward Royzman suggested the existence of four components that make up the bias, which allows us to comprehend in greater detail and depth the way in which this an asymmetry that exists between positives and negative is created.

1. Negative power

Negative power refers to the fact that two events share the same emotional and intensity but have a distinct signification, i.e one is positive, and the other one negative, they don't have the same amount of importance. A negative event is likely to generate more attention than a positive event that has the same amount of intensity and emotionality.

In both cases, Rozin and Royzman believe that this distinction in the acuity of stimuli that are positive and negative is only apparent with respect to situations that have the same level of intensity. If a positive stimulus is associated with an emotional impact far beyond the other stimulus, in this instance, the negative stimulus is likely to be remembered more. the positive stimulus will be better remembered in this scenario.

2. Negative inequality

If an event, be positive or negative and is advancing in space and time and space, the extent in which it is perceived as negative or positive is distinct. An event that is negative will be less positive as it gets closer to an event that is positive.

To understand this better: Let's consider two scenarios with the same level of intensity. The starting of the academic year thought of as negative, and the conclusion of the school year, viewed positively. As the start of the school year gets closer, the event becomes increasingly viewed as far more negative than the conclusion of the course that is viewed as something more positive, but not as significantly.

3. Negative domain

The negative domain is the possibility that the combination of negative and positive aspects result in something negative than what it would be.

The whole is far less positive than its parts, even though there is something positive in these pieces.

4. Negative differentiation

Negative distinction refers to the way people view negativity in a more complicated way than positive.

This isn't a surprise If we attempt to determine the number of words that are part of our vocabulary that have negative connotations. It would be a much longer selection than had we only focused on positive terms.

It has been attempted to offer the evolutionary as well as biological reason that people are more focused on the negative aspects rather than the positive aspects. We will then look at what the biological and evolutionary reasons behind this tendency are.

This can be the reason behind the decision to vote. Many voters are inclined to attach more weight to what the candidate has done and do not vote for him, instead of giving priority to the information about their candidate that proves to be positive.

2. Attention and cognition

Negative information is thought to indicate more movement of brain resources at the cognitive level than positive, as well as having more activity at the cortical levels in which more attention is paid to the negative than positive information.

The negative aspects of someone's attributes, the trauma of incidents, all of these are a magnet for our interest.

People tend to focus more on those concepts that turn out to be negative rather than positive ones, with the vast vocabulary of negative concepts is an illustration of this.

3. Memory and learning

Memory and learning are both an immediate result of the ability to pay attention. The more attention is focused on an incident or event the greater chance it is to be remembered and stored in the memory.

A good example that is not without controversy is the way that punishment puts more weight on memory than reward it.

If someone is punished because they have committed a crime They are more likely to refrain from doing the same thing that has caused harm to them, whereas when they get rewarded for doing something right in the past, they tend be able to overlook it over time.

While this shouldn't be a reason for parents to be more harsh with their children for any reason, it's fascinating to observe how the process of dealing with negative events, such as in this instance, punishment, can have a significant impact on the education of children.

4. Making decisions

The research on negative bias has been focused on how it affects the ability to make decisions, particularly when risk is averted or risk is feared.

In a scenario that a person could either make a profit and lose something else, possible costs, negatives appear to be greater than the potential gains.

The consideration of potential loss and how to avoid them goes along with the idea of negative power as proposed by both Rozin as well as Royzman.

Humans are prone to think about what didn't happen and forget about the positive aspects. Thus, our positive and positive memories are obscured by unpleasant experiences. This is the reason the negativity bias is referring to the importance we attach to the negative.

In addition this is the reason why traumatizing incidents and negative experiences last longer and affect us more than positive experiences. It appears that these events that are more or less unpleasant tend to get more prominent in our thoughts. Let's go deeper.

Many times bad news can have more impact than positive news. In fact, criticism could even have a greater impact on us than compliments.

In his The book The Buddha's Brain, the neuroscientist Rick Hanson ventures an explanation that has been accepted by other researchers regarding the genesis of the evolutionary nature of this negative bias.

According to Hanson the negativity bias is the result of the evolutionary process by our ancestors who learned to make wise choices in extremely risky situations. These kinds of choices are what helped them live long enough to provide for the future generation. They were a matter death and life.

Therefore, those who were in tune with potentially hazardous situations were more likely to endure. In time the brain's structure changed extremely slowly to pay greater focus on negative information rather more than positive information.

Chapter 4: Comprehensive Explanation Of

Dopamine

*The Science Behind Dopamine

Before we get into the details of dopamine-related fasting, we have to comprehend the significance and significance of dopamine in our body. How does it get created? Let's look at the medical aspect that the brain has, which anyone can understand.

The brain of a human is a complex organ. It is home to a variety of processes in the brain, for example, nerve signals and transmissions. Dopamine is released by the brain's area that is known as the Substantia Nigra, which is an area of neurons that is responsible for creating dopamine to the CNS (Central Nervous System) of the human body. The brain is comprised of neurons that are responsible for emitting chemical messages (called neurotransmitters) through their nerve terminals (also known as synapses). They travel to synapses to generate specific signals. Neurotransmitters are released continuously and then absorbed back into the synapses. Thus, the brain can communicate quickly and efficiently.

In the case of dopamine's process within the brain could become extremely complicated to understand, but here's an easy explanation. When this chemical has been released it has to travel to a specific location which is receptors. They take in the dopamine molecule , and are joined together as keys in the lock. This triggers an action in neurons. The message that is sent by the dopamine molecule gets carried to the neuron, and then spreads across the entire nervous system.

When each receptor is full of dopamine molecules and the body is obligated to recycle the dopamine that was not used. This process is known as Reuptake. It can be described as an activity that stabilizes the levels of dopamine and the levels of all other neurotransmitter. Additionally, another process referred to is known as The Negative Feedback Loop which causes too much production of neurotransmitters is stopped.

* The Significance of Dopamine

The problem with the most people is that dopamine receptors of these individuals are destroyed or cease to function which includes the precursors of dopamine. What is the significance of this? In the first place, dopamine comes from an amino acid that is known as Tyrosine. Dopamine is a vital neurotransmitter that plays a variety of roles in the human body. The majority of which are aimed at aiding and supporting the functions that the brain plays. The most important roles include mental focus, emotional state and focus, memory, sleep and movement to mention some. Dopamine is a significant role in sustaining the physical and mental wellbeing of the human body. A healthy level of dopamine in the brain as well as the nervous system can bring benefits like lower cravings, less addiction as well as increased motivation, less levels of depression, less anxiety as well as increased focus and clarity, enhanced sexual life, personal life is healthy and much more.

However low levels of dopamine can affect many people in various ways. Most commonly, the side effects that occur are depression and laziness. People who have lower levels of dopamine will experience less energy and motivation in the course of everyday tasks that they didn't have any difficulties with before. In addition, low levels of dopamine can affect the ability of a person to concentrate on things and make decisions. Also, struggling to lose weight or experiencing coldness are other adverse effects commonly caused by lower levels of dopamine. There are a variety of reasons that can contribute to reducing Dopamine levels within your body including increasing consumption of caffeinated drinks, alcohol and food items, the increase of saturated fats present in fast food, less-quality meat and refined foods like white flour, sugar and bread, elevated stress levels, insufficient sleep unhealthy eating practices, use of drugs as well as a myriad of other similar issues.

* What is Dopamine?

After we've mastered the scientific basis of dopamine, it's time to investigate more deeply into the nature of dopamine and how it functions. Dopamine is linked to feeling great, feeling more pleasure, and an increase in motivation. If dopamine is continuously released within your body, it produces feelings of excitement and joy, which encourages people to participate in activities that produce positive feelings. Dopamine release creates happy and positive feelings in the body.

Dopamine is also known as the "Happy Neurotransmitter It is a deficiency which could cause a number of adverse consequences as described above. Dopamine production in the body has to be at a high amount. A decrease in dopamine neurotransmitter levels are associated with anhedonia-related conditions, in which a person is unable to feel joy in enjoyable activities. In addition, someone with low levels of dopamine is easily distracted and is not connected to other people emotionally. It can also lead to feelings that there is no guilt for certain actions, as well as the inability to feel love. Furthermore, alcohol and drugs addiction can also be the reason for lower levels of dopamine.

However the idea of retail therapy and the thought of buying expensive goods could affect the production of dopamine within the brain, which can create an intense desire and excitement to purchase these products. This could lead to people buying items they desire. This is due to release of dopamine in certain areas within the brain, such as the ventromedial cortex as well as the dztriatum. The mood of a person is improved as dopamine gets released in these areas in the brain. Additionally, the ability of an individual to work and perform at their best is also greatly affected by the production of dopamine.

Additionally, dopamine is associated with pain, and as such it's released when certain types of pain is imposed on the body. When an individual experiences any type of pain your brain produces dopamine in order to shield the body from discomfort. The result of eliminating that pain is to reward the body with satisfaction. The human body is equipped with an reward pathway that is the neural network situated in the center of the brain, which is known as the midbrain. This neural network creates positive and pleasant feelings because of certain actions that increase the survival potential of the human. Dopamine is linked to both pleasure as well as the feeling of pain. If the frontal lobes of the brain experience an increase in levels of dopamine, the degree of pleasure rises while the pain diminishes. Certain people have greater levels of dopamine within their bodies, naturally. This could be because of their genes or a good personality. It could also be due to an excellent diet. Therefore, the individual can handle the discomfort much more easily. Thus, two individuals experiencing the same amount of pain feel it in a different way. Some may feel pain in a heightened way, while another may not feel the pain in any way.

Dopamine is a major part of giving our bodies the feeling of satisfaction, attention, and positive behaviour. Dopamine gives the sensation of joy and inspires people to complete specific tasks. This is why dopamine is commonly referred to as the pleasure system of the brain. It is a result of positive experiences that happen in nature, such as foods, certain substances, and sexual stimulation, including the stimuli connected to them, this is the moment when your body is able to release dopamine. However those with milder illnesses dopamine is found in high amounts in the limbic system in the body which is a collection of brain structures closely linked to emotional and memory issues. There isn't enough dopamine within the cerebral cortex of the brain. This can cause the person to develop an overly paranoid personality. this could lead them to avoid social interaction.

3. Dopamine Fasting How to Know

* What is Dopamine Fasting?

Once we know the basics of dopamine's function and its effects, we can look into the inner workings of dopamine fasting and its advantages. What is dopamine fasting? And why is it so much trend?

The first thing is that people in our society has lost themselves in the ocean of excessive consumption; therefore it has deprives people from pleasure and happiness. This has led to an increased level of depression, low mood, and being less satisfied in general. This all swelled into people seeking out something more to feel happy that is not necessary. Depression, unhappiness, low mood, and a variety of other signs are just the beginning.

Dopamine fasting is involved. If you do this fast it is possible to increase the possibility of recovering the equilibrium within us and bring the sensation of pleasure, joy, as well as happiness to its original place.

* Who is The Best Person to Apply For A Dopamine Fast?

Fasting as a method isn't appropriate for all. Dopamine-based fasting allows the person to have a break from intense dopamine spikes and sensory oversaturation. If you're someone who is dependent on porn, alcohol, drugs social media, or other addictive behaviors, you're in need of taking a dopamine fast. Dopamine fasting can aid in healing and establishing the foundation for your brain's ability to experience happiness and delight every time. If you're an individual who is incredibly committed to achieving your goals, or you simply need to swiftly move on from an unpleasant aspect in your own life doing a dopamine-based fast might be the perfect solution to your issues.

* Duration Of A Dopamine Fast

Dopamine fasting is quite amazing and is a must to try. It actually works and isn't a gimmick that will make you feel deprived of your most beloved pleasures. If you begin to feel like your addiction has taken over your life, and is causing you to neglect your duties this is the time that dopamine-based fasting should be considered. The dopamine-induced fast can last for several hours, or for all week. You could fast for up to up to 24 hours to restore the dopamine receptors in your body and feel that you feel differently. Also, with a doctor's guidance, you have the option of fasting for a longer duration of duration. The length of time will vary for each person based on the degree of addiction. Every person who has an dopamine-induced fast must follow their individual needs as well as keeping their health under control. This is the same for repeated fasts. If you think you'll have to repeat the dopamine-induced fast for the second or third time, be sure that you're fit enough to be able to do the task.

* Can A Dopamine Fast Be Harmful?

It's not just the practice of fasting that causes harm it is the addiction itself that could be fatal for your body and mind. It is essential to keep the proper amount and level of dopamine within one's system. Thus, someone who is attempting the dopamine speed will certainly be able to achieve the results they are looking to achieve and will create a perfect equilibrium in their lives.

* The Latest Trends In Dopamine Fasting

In recent time, various forms of fasting has become more popular, be it an intermittent or cleanse fasting. Dopamine-based fasting has also been hopping on the fasting bandwagon and with a justifiable reason. Human desires have become the focus of our mind and we've become addicted to things that elevate addiction to a new level. Be it social media, smothering yourself with alcohol, food, drugs shopping, the latest technologies and everything else has bombarded our mind with high doses of dopamine. Dopamine fasting advocates have said that in order to attain the right amount of dopamine within the body and avoid extreme addiction doing dopamine fasting is the option.

When you are on a dopamine high the sense of focus and clarity is restored to you. If your mind isn't being continuously stimulated and clouded, you will see the brain returning to its independence and ability to think. Without interference from electronic devices or sexual activity, or any other kind of addiction, one is able to achieve their goals and again. Dopamine fasting is the hottest new trend available for all to experience.

4. The Signs that Show You're in need of Dopamine Fasting

Imagine this. What you believed you thought you knew about your life has changed due to the way you conduct yourself. Your dependence on your smartphone or drugs or any other issues make you feel empty in your life, uninterested, vulnerable and very lonely in your life. It is difficult to know what to do, and every second of time seems to be a long time. Your bed is stained in crying as you sit in bed thinking what you have done with your life. The next morning you're required to get yourself out of bed and walk around with a an unnatural smile at your face, wondering what you can do to fix this. Do you feel this is similar to your own life? Do you see any similarities to yours? If you answered yes then, my dear friend, you're seeking a dose of dopamine speedy.

It can be emotionally draining If you aren't aware of how to manage it. Your life can turn upside down and be affected in a negative way. If you do not take care to control it this can lead to ruining your relationships and sending you to the path of depression. Here are some of the typical indicators to watch out for to tell you that you're in the need of a dopamine boost fast.

Chapter 5: Benefits Of Meditative, Yoga, And

Other Activities During A Dopamine Fast

Exercise has been proven to boost the release of dopamine receptors within your brain. Furthermore, research suggests that high-intensity interval exercise (HIIT) is very effective in this particular region. For instance, in the sprinting workout it is possible to run for about 15 to 20 seconds and then rest to allow a sufficient recuperation time. The rest time is different for each person. Some people will be fine to rest for 30 seconds, while others require 2 or 3 minutes. Therefore, you must take a break until you feel adequate to continue with full force. Repeat this method until you've had approximately 4-8 sprints. You can also perform the HIIT program on a stationary bike or similar device which allows you to get a high output. If you'd rather running a jog or slower run, that's okay too. It's a fact that regular exercise helps your body to produce more dopamine.

* Yoga and Meditation

If you are meditating by using a technique, you attempt to let yourself relax. It is known as a mind to body medicine that highly affects the psychoneuroimmunology of a human. It recommends that you exercise controlling your senses. Your senses of smell, sight, taste, sound, and even touch must be in your control. In addition, body movement is a crucial factor. These factors influence the function in your central nervous system the autonomic nervous system peripheral nervous system, the limbic system, cardiovascular system and immune system. These body systems are accountable for controlling the human body's behaviour and emotions. There is no doubt about it that when the body and mind have synchronized, the final outcome will be the perfect balance of cell and nerve. Additionally, you can get similar results through running, jogging, or running. These activities all give you satisfaction.

According to research, when you begin to regularly meditate the release of dopamine is increased by 65percent. The nervous system undergoes an ongoing change as a result of the continual stimulation that is triggered by regular meditation. Neurotransmitters and neuromodulators could trigger the production of dormant or unused neurons to create these. Additionally, the new plasticity and new connections may be created by the brain. This could result in the brain thinking, rationalizing as well as reacting in a manner that is different from our body's inputs to sensory opposed to what is typically expected.

So, when you have committed to meditation the frontal cortex of your brain lights up. It is an part within the brain in front of the forehead. The limbic system is then put working and is an intricate system of nerves and networks inside the brain. It regulates a person's primary desires and emotions. So, when you settle down with the proper intention to meditate your thoughts, emotions play their part and you feel more optimistic.

Additionally, various types of meditation have proved their effectiveness for people with anxiety problems. It has been proven that meditation can greatly aid in producing dopamine. However, there's a second chemical that is responsible for the sensation of pleasure and happiness known as serotonin. It is also released through meditation. This release aids in improving concentration and imagination. Additionally, meditation can help people feel calm and have an inner tranquility. Thus, doing these exercises while on your dopamine fast can significantly improve your life and enhance your creativity.

Chapter 6: What Are The Do's And Don'ts Of

Dopamine Fasting

* Food and Your Body's release of Dopamine

Before we dive deep into the specifics of what's allowed during a dopamine-free fast, we should begin by focusing on food and the way it can affect your body's levels of dopamine. When it concerns food, it can greatly impact an individual's mood. It can make you feel depressed and unmotivated, or leave you feeling full of happiness, energy, excitement, less stress and generally feeling happier.

There are several general categories of food which affect the mood of an individual in different ways, such as probiotics. The human digestive tract is thought to be the second brain. Therefore, taking care of the health of your digestive tract will lead to more positive brain. Therefore, the food you eat should contain some kind of probiotic. This will lead to an improved immune system, better digestion, and an overall sensation of happiness.

The second category is vegetables and fruits. Most people will grab the orange or a banana but there are many other innovative options to choose from. For instance, it's possible to add vegetables to baking, like carrot muffins. Studies suggest that eating more fruits and vegetables will give you not just more energy, as well as a feeling of peace and joy. So, it is suggested to consume seven servings of fruits and vegetables every throughout the day. Fruits and vegetables are packed with antioxidants and flavonols. consequently, once someone takes in and nourish their body with foods like these that are full of nutrients, their bodies respond by generating feelings of joy and energy. This is better to choose apples or oranges.

In addition, everyone likes being in a good mood, as it gives them the feeling of being happy. There are a myriad of food items one can consume to boost dopamine levels within the brain. Apart from food, having more sun exposure on the skin can also be beneficial since it increases the creation of Vitamin D and lower stress. Be aware when you are in the sun. Do not stay for an extended duration. A few minutes of exposure to the sun is sufficient.

Additionally, eating a large amount of leafy greens and raw veggies is a fantastic method to improve your overall health. They supply your body with vitamins as well as the minerals required in aiding the brain, and include the lower risk of developing mental illnesses. Also, it is recommended to limit the consumption of beverages that contain caffeine since they could cause people to crash as a result of over stimulation to the brain. In addition, having a good night's sleep plays a crucial part in maintaining a healthy state of mind, which includes the dopamine production in the body.

* Things Permitted, and Not Permitted, During Dopamine Fast

Fasting in is a reference to abstaining either from eating or engaging in other activities. In the case of dopamine-free fasting, the basic principle is to abstain from any enjoyable activity you can and to aim at discomfort. It is possible to do this for at least 24 hours, or for up to seven days. If it's your first time trying the dopamine-based fast, it is recommended to try it over the weekend.

Let's look at the things that are and are not permitted during a dopamine fast. Here is a checklist that you must read through to know what you can and should not do during the dopamine fast.

DO NOT USE DOPAMINE EASY:

1. Do not entertain thoughts of sexuality or engage in any sexual activities.

2. Avoid eating any food.

3. Do not consume any medication.

4. Avoid using the internet or your mobile phone.

5. Avoid participating in any conversations with other people as they are considered as stimulating and fun.

6. Don't take hot showers.

7. Don't do any reading.

8. Avoid doing any strenuous exercise.

9. Avoid listening at any kind of music.

DO'S OF DOPAMINE Fasting:

1. Take part in prayer or meditation.

2. Keep a diary and note down all thoughts and thoughts you've had during your fasting

journey. The ability to reflect on your thoughts is crucial.

3. Take a cold shower.

4. Do take a walk in the sun and catch some sun.

5. Take part in a gentle exercise.

6. Make sure you drink only water.

If you're planning to perform your dopamine-free diet for a month or more than one week, then the only food that you must consume is organic foods. It should be sufficient to last you the duration. Also, it's essential to find a peaceful area without distractions and pay attention to your surroundings. Soon, you will start to notice chemicals taking effects in your brain. And your insights will show up also. The entire journey of your mind is an unforgettable experience.

Chapter 7: Dopamine Fast Challenge

Dopamine fasts are something you can do for yourself and your personal growth. So, it is advised not to join any of your friends to participate in this challenge. Instead, you should take it on by yourself for your own personal benefit. Every person is unique, therefore each person is trying to do something different by completing this fasting challenge. We are now moving to the dopamine fast challenge.

Nowadays, everyone is busy with their mobile phones. Everywhere you go, you will find people with their phones in their hands , and are completely immersed in whatever it is they're doing. It doesn't matter if they are texting or talking while driving or walking or in restaurants or at the library, or shopping, the reliance on the phone has risen to a new level. Many people don't pay enough attention when they order food at a restaurant since they're too distracted by their mobile phones. This is because humans have lost sight of their basic needs and gotten involved in activities that have little worth to their lives and causes them to be distracted. If you are experiencing this issue, Dopamine fasting could be the ideal choice for you.

Dopamine-induced excitement causes you to think about your past, present and the future. It allows you to aware of what you feel inside, without the influence of others. Additionally, you realize that you have to rely entirely on your own judgment when it comes to your choices in your life. In this instance it is not your age that have any bearing on your decisions. Therefore doing a dopamine-based fast can be beneficial and educational for anyone who tries it. It is the perfect moment to analyze your thoughts examine your ideas, and discover what makes you happy and what isn't.

A lot of times individuals don't have the time they need to be at home and contemplate deeply about the things they do and how their lives are. They generally rely on the perceptions of others about what they're like as individuals, whether they are friends, teachers family members, or even the media. In the beginning you're dependent on the parents of your children, close relatives, as well as your acquaintances when it comes to thinking about your purpose in life. But, you will reach a point that you'll need to take back control of the way you think and create an ideal life plan which only you are able to create. This is all possible as you go through an intense dopamine rush, and your mind is clear free of all the chaos in your life.

Everybody believes it's essential to stay in contact with people you know so people use their phones as opposed to other activities. Although, it's vital to be in contact with everyone, talk to them or browse the web and so on. But if you keep doing this over and over again, it will have its effects. Additionally, it's very unfortunate that this behavior is also addictive and that's one of the reasons that drives you to dopamine-freezing in order to better understand the brain. When you realize that you're doing what's good for yourself this creates a sense of confidence in you , which gives you a sense of satisfaction. When you begin doing dopamine-based fasts, you will be capable of achieving fulfillment in your life according to what you desire.

Additionally, you don't require to be an experienced yoga instructor or be a single person for an effective dopamine-fueled quick. But planning it out ahead of time will certainly be beneficial. It will help you check the way things are going for you and also answer some questions regarding your life. For instance:

* Am I pleased with the improvements I've achieved in the course I am currently

* Am I meeting the demands of the class and earning my desired grade?

Are I making enough money to be happy?

Are I happy with my present social life?

Are I physically fit to compete in the cycling race which is set to begin?

If you can answer these questions honestly and with a sense of reality you'll be able to understand the current state that you have planned for your future. You'll be able to determine how and when you should change things and it's your job to implement the modifications. There will come a point in your life that it is essential to make changes. Like a car, which must be maintained to enhance it's performance, so should an individual's life, but it's a more critical circumstance.

Thus, making yourself do the dopamine high can give you the chance you'll need to think clearly about your life's purpose and goals. Do not listen to radio or music and avoid talking to any person on your mobile. Don't just do nothing. Utilize this time to think of new concepts, come up with fresh ideas and be happy about what you're doing and trying to achieve since you're finally taking note of your own life. Make the most of this time to be grateful for your life and take in the natural beauty. You could go canoeing, hiking or meditate for a walk. It is your choice. Be sure to be completely alone during the dopamine fasting trip.

Chapter 8: How To Stay Motivated And Keep

From Stopping Your Dopamine Quickly

Dopamine fasting is the ideal method to improve your health, mentally, emotionally or physically. But, in our fast-paced lifestyle it is often challenging for people who aren't used to it when they are trying to change their routines and habits of fasting. It is also quite scary. If this is your first time it is recommended to test the dopamine intermittent fast of 24 hours. Whatever way you choose, this method of fasting is extremely beneficial to your healthof the body, and it's not any cost and you can perform it with ease. It is suggested to incorporate this practice as a regular one to your diet.

In addition, the effects of fasting are distinct from person to person. Some may feel more energetic, and others may feel hazy. This is why it is crucial to not get carried away in this. That's why it's advised to keep a diary throughout your fasting times. Write in it in as much detail as you can during your fasting period. Journal entries should include the date, date, and the time of days that you're

135

fasting. While doing a dopamine fast, the individual's personality is revealed. As such it is likely that you'll have moments of insight and inspiration when you write your journal. This is why you should not be averse to this great chance and keep a journal as long as you can during the duration of your dopamine fast.

It is easier to be motivated to keep going on a fast if you have goals or a vision that you set for yourself before starting your journey to fast. If you're looking to experience the success you desire during your dopamine fasting experience, staying motivated is vital. Your desire to achieve what you'd like to accomplish at the end of the day is the primary source for your determination. If you're not willing to see a positive change to your lifestyle, then you most likely won't stick with the program; it's straightforward as this. This principle applies to everything you desire in your life. If you're truly committed to something, you'll want to accomplish whatever it is. Furthermore, if you're determined to map out every step you must take to accomplish your goals and succeed, then the success is definitely yours. There's nothing in the world that can hinder an extremely motivated person who wants to be successful.

* Motivation

The most important factor you require to keep your motivation high is concentration. When you're focused upon your objective, your brain is able to focus on trying to accomplish it. It reveals the drive of an individual and aids to achieve success. It's not rocket science, and it is simple once one realizes all they require is concentrate in order to achieve success. Thus, you have to be extremely focused to attain the top of your game when you're experiencing a high-dopamine rush.

* Discipline

Discipline can be described as rules you need to observe. Discipline in the life of a person is similar to the boat that isn't equipped with an control. It is impossible to develop without discipline in their lives. You must be extremely disciplined to be able to endure an intense dopamine-fueled fast. When you're in the dopamine high and you are in a dopamine high, the distractions around you are likely to tempt you. However you have to remain disciplined enough to stay clear of these temptations and continue in order to return to your normal life.

Additionally, it is essential to plan ahead when it comes time when you need to end your fast. This is an essential step during the whole process. If you're not prepared before the time, the craving can result in overeating, which could cause stomach damage and discomfort. When the fast is over you must remember that your body has just gone through an energizing and rejuvenating journey. Avoid food items that are loaded with sugars, carbohydrates, or other ingredients. Also, avoid alcohol, soda and milk (you can choose to have low-fat or fat-free varieties).

Chapter 9: Definition Of Negativity

Thinking About Thoughts

Have you ever thought about how thought processes function within our brains? How does the brain of a human evolve to think of thoughts? What purpose serves it?

From the moment we are born, and before that our minds are always thinking. It is a task that is intrinsic to the human. While we all are born with the capacity to think but focused work is essential to be able to think to ensure that it is able to reach the highest levels. It is not restricted to an automatic process. If it wasn't for this, we'd have no or little awareness.

Perkins in 1998 says how the brains of infants develop within a framework of thought. This means that by the time they become adulthood they can be observant and deal with difficult situations. This includes organizing their time and developing a sound approach to life, to comprehend the viewpoint of another , to be critical of their views and find a way out when the situation seems to be insurmountable and to recognize and deal with rumors that are not true.

Research conducted in Project Zero's Project Zero team shows that the majority of people are not equipped with the necessary thinking abilities, attitudes, and alerts. They are passively indifferent situations that provoke thought. They are not sensitive to signs that prompt thought. They don't cultivate the thoughts of deep reflection that include: Asking questions about the facts, look over the obvious discover the unspoken side of things or think differently for a moment and take advantage of all thinking-provoking opportunities.

Therefore, youngsters and children have to be taught these behaviors, skills and triggers of the mind, but they are not able to develop them spontaneously.

One reason we do not have awareness of the thoughts we think is because either way, our thoughts aren't visible to those who surround us. In many cases circumstances that trigger them aren't even noticed.

In the realm of education the ability to record the object of learning using our senses can greatly aid in the learning process. For instance when a child learns to write seeing the various lyrics can help you to remember the words.

For high school students who is studying a cell, when they are able to view cells under microscopes, they can more easily construct creating a mental image, and it is used in conjunction with the creation of concepts for example, a child trying to learn to play music with an instrument, through listening to the performance.

With the help of a professional musician, you can get an idea of the rhythm you will have to perform. The learning process can profoundly affects perceptions Learning objectives: The observation of learning goals:

The mind is completely invisible. Most times thoughts, they are hidden in the underside of the amazing motor of our brain. Luckily, neither the thought as well as the opportunities to think need to necessarily be hidden as often they are.

Indirectly or directly It allows us to replicate, imitate or evoke, alter and alter that perception, and to develop our knowledge, which is personal to us. The issue is when the goal of learning is considered as a thing in itself, since the subject of study is inaccessible, at the very most in the beginning and the contexts that trigger it.

Everything "Negativity"

My friend is an amazing artist and illustrator. I can assure you that she is among the finest I've seen, and I'm a person with an education in art. Today, she has an active account on Instagram Creator that showcases her work, as well as growing her social media profile for her work as an artist. She is now a bit agitated over the slow process of growing her profile from nothing to a successful.

In addition She recently followed a famous artist who is a blue tick Instagram prodigy , whose timeline gives an incredible visual experience. If you're an artist, you should try to be like them. This artist initiated a trend that prompted the other artist on Instagram to follow in his footsteps. The trend grew into an extremely successful hashtag that was followed by posts in the hundreds of thousands.

Naturally, my beloved was intrigued to join in the trend. She was enticed by the chance to increase her reach, gain more attention and be followed, watched and republished by the person who started the trend. A mere 24 hours later I am more excited than she's ever been before in the year 2020. She posted the image she had created as part the trend, and was expecting to explode - but positively and, naturally.

The next thing I notice I received a string of text messages while I was walking towards my Uber to return homethat evening. It turns out that she didn't get enough interaction than she thought she would. She was able to scan the biography that of an artist began the trend, and was constantly mulling over the inclusions to other artist in the narratives. The other artists weren't as good, at least that's what I've heard.

Two hours had passed and she was in complete silence. In her bedroom. In her room. Instagram. and her profile on the artist. Reposts and shares in stories been halted. It felt as if the ship had sailed and we were a bit late to get to the dock.

At this point she was convinced she wasn't good enough, and that her work didn't make an impact. I was in a rush to free her of that funk by continuously telling her about the great work she had achieved with the Procreate canvas that she had created on her iPad. I wanted to shout at the roof of my head so that people like Sandro Botticelli would hear me and understand my thoughts.

However, she wasn't at all this time. She showed me hundreds of profiles which had been shared and had higher engagement. She insisted that she wasn't adequate enough. It was an hour and she was analysing what had gone wrong, constantly critiquing her artand simply pointing out things that were not in line with her work.

The result was that I observed her practicing other styles. She looked up a lot of styles that were quite different to hers, and then started to study. If she were Renaissance She was attempting the Manga world Manga in the present. It was an ideal recipe for catastrophe.

The night went by and we awoke with the exact same conversation as well as her angry face. Her beauty was still there and, let's face it, she was pretty. However, it was the beginning of sadness. She once more went through Instagram but without success. If there was a sign of hope, it's been lost.

After an hour after showering, I was struggling to figure out what I could do to improve the situation? Perhaps she could be paid for her project to increase her reach on Instagram? I was putting the pieces back in their the right place when I heard knocks at the bathroom door. Naturally I recognized the sequence of knocks.

Then, I realize she walked into the bathroom, and then drew my curtains as if I were Venus in the painting of our Boticelli friend's "Mars as well as Venus". I was thinking that Oscar (my canine) had puked once more. It was actually the iPhone and my blurred vision, trying to understand what she was showing me.

Good news! the artist posted her work, enjoyed itand even wrote a comment on the post. She was thrilled and I'll tell you that was more, he thoroughly admired her work. In reminiscing about this personal incident I began to think about how our brains work and in what way is the human brain vulnerable for negative thought patterns.

Never again have I heard her discussing altering her style or criticizing her work in a negative way.

If we don't define the term "negativity" and without defining the term "negativity", we can be able to find many examples of negative people. The person that pops into your mind would be the person who is looking at"the "glass half-empty" and who doesn't end having a good feeling about any situation, and then when situations change and they believe that things is going to get better They claim that they were more fortunate before. It is tiring to hear it however, it's that person who is experiencing the worst experience. Their life is over.

There are many kinds of people who are negative. They may only be able to whine, but not listen or considering possibilities for solutions. The contestants who are participating in "the long-distance race against negativity" will be always going be worse than you are, either due to their bad luck or because their experiences were more severe.

Then there are the "chronic" adverses the ones who think constantly about their luck, their issues or their unjust situation and for whom there is no relief.

It is also easy to get caught in the pit of negativity. Every one of us puts ourselves in the shoes of the victim, blaming others and not seeking solutions. A psychologist named Stephen Karpman developed in 1968 what was known as"the "Dramatic Triangle."

In it, he points out that often we play this victim role because that is the situation we were in or chose to live in the world we live in, where there were rescuers (who even assisted and helped without having to ask for assistance) as well as persecutors (always seeking someone to criticize or punish). Even if this is the way we are used to functioning, and , in reality it works but it's not a sustainable way of coping.

Neuropsychologists have studied negativity. Their research suggests that, as our brains work through neural networks, when we are prone to repetitive thoughts about something in particular it will learn to "activate" the same neurons in response to thoughts, feelings , or experiences that are similar.

Also, if we constantly hold negative or even victimizing thoughts Our minds will be able to connect with these networks whenever we are with similar experiences.

If, for instance, I fall and my cell phone is damaged If I'm constantly thinking about my unfortunate luck then my brain will start thinking of the kind "why is it that this happens to me! " But not "well it's so old , I'd need to make changes soon". It's a sign that negativity causes us to become ever more negative.

Positive psychology warns us that our mind has an inexplicably strong attraction to negative thoughts. It was first introduced in the 1990s in the 1990s by Martin Seligman and continued by Mihaly Csikszentmihalyi who is not and also the extremely insightful Jonathan Haidt, it focuses on the research of psychological health and various positive aspects of laughter and creativity to happiness or wisdom itself.

This field of psychology is the opposite of a long-standing history centered on studying the neuronal causes as well as the potential remedies for anxiety, depression stress, and other mental illnesses and demons. It is a quest to discover and promote positive behavior when faced with the reality that the negative and threatening can be a part of your mind, and it is much stronger than the positive. The negative bias, sets us up for both good and bad.

148

We'll get into the negativity bias in the future in greater depth. However, for the moment this bias to negativity could be seen as a biological drag. It is a perfect fit for evolutionary reasons. The automatic brain hyperresponsiveness (faster than conscious decision-making) is what lets us save our lives from every possible danger. However, these can be false alarms (for instance, when we slam into the chair prior to the sudden appearance in a film of a knife, or a snake, or we move the path when an unknown person approaches at night).

The brain is not equipped with the same system of reactivity to the good and pleasing, since the world isn't about it. The fact that negativity is more dominant than the positive in the mind is the reason why the pain of a loss in an economy more than the joy of an improvement and also the feelings that negative news triggers can be more intense.

The Swedish epidemiologist Hans Rosling, famous for his amazing TED talks that include statistics about the development of nations and their progress, has been studying for years the inaccurate negative perception that Westerners hold of the developing world.

Most people believe that all over the world there are more deaths due to violence as well as fewer girls going to schools, lower rates of vaccination as well as limited access to electricity, the Internet as well as more species threatened with disappearing ... that there are actually. This is a belief he attributes to the innate feeling of negativeness, as he refers to"the" lack of awareness of our past, the notion that, even though things aren't perfect it is immoral to accept that they improve and to the deceitful image that is propagated by the media and the activists.

Rosling's negative instinct and the negative tendencies of positive psychologists are a reference to the same finding in neuroscience. In the background of this knowledge is science there's certainly a lot of pop psychology that has the ability to alter the truth and create self-help products with greater or lesser scientific basis however, this doesn't negate the factual existence of this quick, determined and instinctual human reaction to the most negative and bad news.

Like everything else in the human race There is an enormous variance between individuals on the scale of optimism-pessimism which is a genetic foundation (this is the reason why Jonathan Haidt calls the "cortical lottery" which refers towards the cortex in the front). In the current time of a epidemics, we are able to recognize not only the degree the negative bias is evident but also the range of reactions between individuals.

Positive Cycles Thinking

There are two kinds of thoughts: positive and negative. Both go through a process that feeds them. as the cycle progresses or takes place it gains strength. When it is fed by the negative energies, it draws on greater strength, and the human being is the one that lets it continue its cycle since this is where the brain creates the thoughts.

If we consider negative thoughts prior to the "X" scenario what is the outcome? Absolutely that we will have negative results because we have a tendency to program our minds to get these results. If we view motivation as unattainable and we don't think we can be able to achieve much and will always fail in difficult situations. Maybe we concentrate on the mistake, on the words they'll say, on our anxieties or anxieties. We let them control us, instead of us governing them.

A study in psychology found that the average person is able to have around 4000 thoughts per day. out of those 30% are negative while the remainder are routine thoughts. A majority of people are caught in a negative thought cycle without realizing that they can get out from this vicious cycle.

What is the reason why it seem like our brains evolved to help us think in this way?

Repetitive and negative thinking are logical in the context of evolution in biology, since our ancestors had to use this regular thinking to manage the everyday activities of the day life. Negative thinking was a way to constantly be looking for natural disasters or predators.

Your great fantastic amazing fantastic, great grandpa determined that it was best to eat all the wild boar he hunted just before wolves began to circle in the area.

It is the brain's design to generate beta waves in survival situations However, beta waves are those that define the thoughts of stress or fear. Fear is what made our ancestors to survive. Fear was what made your great - let's just stick and let your grandfather live to fight another day against wolves.

While we're no longer living in the wild seeking to avoid predators Our brains continue to operate as if we lived in those circumstances.

If we awake in the morning, our brains have been in the delta and theta as we slept however, the brain immediately shifts to beta. Then, as we're running in the late hour, and we begin to fret about the tasks we need to accomplish during the day, or about the presentation we need to complete in the next couple of hours. We begin to be worried and the evolution mechanism previously employed to recognize predators is activated.

Prior to leaving home our brains are flooded with anxiety-inducing thoughts. These kinds of thoughts, or what's known as "the mind of the caveman" can have a negative impact on our bodies.

Thoughts Are Things

In the study of 68,222 adult anxiety was found to increase the risk of dying by 20%.

The same skill that made our ancestors able to survive is what kills many people in the present. Our minds have become an enemy to our survival.

Our minds are like an unlit room in which photographs are made. It is the location where our life takes shape.

What we really are isn't the name we use, or our appearance, or what we wear, or our families, or the vehicle we drive in or the location in which we reside. What we are is the beliefs that are shaped in this dark space.

The subconscious mind is completely non-judgmental and doesn't decide the truth of a belief or habit is beneficial or not. Because of this, it is normal to be constantly surprised by the variety of negative thoughts or images are in our minds that are reflected through our everyday life experiences repeatedly and over. It is rare that we encounter a situation which we didn't create within our minds.

To make a difference in the world, we have to change the dark space. If you believe in this idea of your subconscious as being a dark space and you be able to see that the process of changing your life doesn't need to be a complicated process. Instead, it's simply changing the image that is appearing in this dark space.

You'll be amazed to learn that all the attitudes and beliefs that you learned and embraced in your early years are the beliefs which have the greatest impact and power in your present life.

We all have these images generated by ideas and beliefs that we've completely lost, yet are lurking in the dark recesses of our thoughts. This demonstrates how important it is to choose your mental images and thoughts carefully.

For instance, if you believe that if someone near you sneezes , you'll be sick, that belief is the thought in your mind which generates your expectations. The next time someone else next to you sneezes, it is likely that you will become sick.

And, on the other hand what do you think that miracle cures originate? They also originate from our subconscious minds.

If you can fill the dark space with truths, then your external world will reflect the reflection of the inner images that speak truth.

The subconscious mind recognizes these realities and then immediately begins to repair your body. Not only heals but also wealth creation happens in the subconscious mind. And it is crucial to increase the wealth of the subconscious before you begin to see abundance within your own life.

Health and illness are the result of our dominating mental and spiritual states.

A sudden emotional trauma and a mind brimming with anxiety, can trigger heart issues. Doctors are now beginning to acknowledge the fact that under stress and emotional tension, and especially in the midst of anger blood is able to create a chemical build-up in the ligaments of the body.

Anger, fear, anxiety, jealousy, and other mental issues are all mental and are the hidden reason behind the majority of today's most prevalent physical ailments and issues.

A healthy mind shows in a healthy physique, and similarly an unhealthy mental state manifests in a physical problem. The mind is a literal thing!

Modern psychology confirms that all thoughts and feelings we've had the pleasure of experiencing and thinking about as conscious are stored in our subconscious minds and are active and manifest subconsciously as tendencies that form the body's condition in health or illness and affect our reactions to life and to various experiences.

It does not mean that the disease was caused by a particular idea, but rather is the result from an imbalance within the mind. Many suffer from anguish as well as emotional pain violent outbursts from anger and resentment, intense rage anxiety and other mental states where there was no particular idea. The most important thing to remember is that the activities of the mind creates an inverse physical and emotionally unbalanced state. is always a cause for unhygienic physical and mental conditions that can be detrimental to your body and in the life.

Thoughts are real that have the ability to manifest into physical matterand are the reason for every condition.

The majority of us are living in a world of routine which offers us peace and security. The prior plan of work outlines the direction we need to take. When we run into restrictions, we get trapped in thoughts that are not spontaneous and for the greater part, limits our imagination. This are, in turn, worse with time.

Rumination: Bottleneck in the Negativity Cycle

Human beings are naturally inclined to organize and plan our actions. This provides us with assurance and security. However, it restricts other essential aspects of our lives, creativity and spontaneity can be distinct.

So, as we can see negative and obsessive thoughts that humans have are several factors that affect the quality of our lives. One of the most common is the rumination. It occurs when our thoughts remain connected to an aspect that may be imaginary or real and as a result causes extreme stress and discomfort.

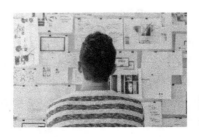

Unaware of it the first time, we begin an endless cycle of stress in which we are prompted by any negative thought or worry We become accustomed to feeling uncomfortable and the discomfort increases with the course of.

In this manner, we are unable to focus, and it becomes more difficult to handle positive thoughts because we tend to attach all our thoughts to the specific events we are aware of that could trigger negative emotions. This loop doesn't enable us to release our minds from the burden of stress.

This article outlines the connections with the processes of cognitive processing associated with negative attitude towards the problem such as concern and rumination. and depressive, anxious symptoms, and the current one of eating disorder problems.

Negative problems and worry about the future are transdiagnostic causes for agoraphobia and panic symptoms or generalized anxiety disorder the fear of social interaction and behavior eating while brooding is an indicator of depression as well as posttraumatic stress disorder. eating disorders that cause behavioral. The reflection process is linked to social fear. The results are discussed in relation to the theory of social phobia as well as stress post-traumatic.

The recurring negative thoughts are thought of as indicators of cognitive vulnerability to various mood, anxiety, and behavioral disorders. These are those that involve an alert constant, continuous, and frequent mental activity that is involuntary, that concentrate on negative aspects of oneself and the world.

Rumination, particularly is a predictor of the onset of depression. It plays an important role in the maintenance of depression and its repeat incidence.

Rumination can be described as a repetitive pattern of thoughts and actions that center your attention on yourself, depression, symptoms along with their causes the meanings and effects of these signs, instead of focusing on solutions to the causes of these symptoms.

Many studies view rumination as an entity that has two dimensions, that is characterized by two components reflective, which are described as a process of reflection which is intended to engage in solving cognitive problems to ease the symptoms of depressed mood. Then there are the reproaches, that consist of self-reproachful or negative rumination and situations that are compared passively the current situation with a standards that have not been met.

Apart from thinking about it, another negative thoughts that repeat is the worry thought it is an ongoing chain of thought or verbal language images (although not necessarily the first) filled with negative emotions and largely inexplicably difficult to control. The process of worrying is the attempt to solve a mental issue the issue, whose resolution is unclear. It also comes with the risk of having one or more negative outcomes.

So, worry is closely connected to the process of fear. As with rumination, worry is the most prominent aspect of generalized anxiety disorders. But, it's also frequent with other anxiety disorders and mood disorders.

A mental process that is associated with the two processes of worry and rumination can be described as a negative attitude towards the issue that is described as "a belief system which reflect the view of a challenge as an obstacle to wellbeing and expressing doubts about the capacity to deal with problems, and the tendency to become skeptical about the outcome". When a group of people are sampled with negative attitudes it is shown to be a factor in depression.

If we consider gender as a factor, women are twice more likely than males to develop depression. The distinctions that become apparent during adolescence and into adulthood, but in the older population there are no distinctions with regard to the severity of depression with regard to gender.

However the higher rate of depression among women has been analyzed considering a range of theories, one of which is responding styles theory which suggests that women have a more introspective style than men. This is why they are more prone to depression. In this way there are more reproaches for women, and they are also more likely to score higher for depression, negative attitudes towards issues and criticisms.

Obsessive thoughts: The Dangers of Rumination

It is normal to take a moment and think about the painful events or worries of our day. We hope to discover a new perspective that lessens our burden and lets us advance. However, this process of self-reflection can go wrong. Instead of experiencing the emotional relief we need, we replay the same painful scenes in our heads every time and feel more sad angry, frustrated, or sad.

We replay the events of a bitter breakup, and then re-examine the subtleties of that final conversation. We replay in our heads each and every detail of the final moments before we were impacted by loss or trauma. We replay every meeting in which our boss made a snide comment before our coworkers or we practiced different ways of dealing with a dispute or discussion that didn't conclude as we'd would have liked.

The need to reflect on our worries could happen anytime and take up our thoughts while we are to the store, bathing, as we're cooking dinner, or even when we're trying to complete the work. In a flash our mental state is already in chaos and our emotions are more swollen than ever before.

The Hidden Risks of Being Involved in the Ruminative Cycle

Rumination is regarded as a non-adaptive method of self-reflection because it can provide new insight but only increases the psychological and emotional stress we feel. It is obvious that ruminative patterns are stressful, but what's less evident are the serious dangers they can pose to our physical and mental health.

Ruminations can create an unending loop that could be a trap for us. The urge to think can be addictive, and the more we think about it in our mind, the more we are attracted to do it.

* Rumination increases the likelihood of developing depression, as well as prolonging the time between depression episodes.

* It's linked to an increased risk of misuse. It is common to drink when we are at the edge of sadness and irritability due to our constant contemplations.

* This phenomenon is linked with a higher chance of developing eating disorders. A lot of us rely on food to cope with the stressful feelings that our reflections cause.

* It can trigger negative thoughts. The fact that we spend a lot of time thinking about unpleasant and difficult events can influence our overall perceptions in a manner that we start to see the world around us negatively , too.

Additionally, it promotes the delay of solving issues. In the case of women with ruminative tendencies discover a lump on their breasts take two months longer than those with no such tendency to book an exam with a doctor. A study has confirmed that.

* Having thoughts that cause ruminations enhances our reactions to physiological and psychological stress in a manner that the risk of developing cardiovascular diseases increase.

The straightforward and basic idea of thinking is the process of thinking, imagining and articulating ideas and images within the human mind. Based on the favorable approach, whether pleasant or not of the thought, it can are classified as either positive or negative, and the consequent effect on the daily life of every one of us as an individual and as a group.

The existence of both schools of thought have always been considered. An infinite variety of religious, philosophical and psychological trends have been addressing their studies and their implications in a collective way and.

It has been recent times that there was increasing concern about these issues that led to their increased distribution both through media and science in order to spread more extensive knowledge base, that provides greater clarity and depth the impact they provide to the various kinds of thoughts that influence the well-being of the human body, and the formation of inter-personal bonds.

Negative thoughts can trigger anxiety, stress, and fear. They can also cause us to feel a lot of psychological discomfort and can seriously affect our mental well-being.

When we are able to recall, our brains begin to flood our minds with all sorts of thoughts and ideas. This is not just positive since it allows us to develop the creative and cognitive section of our brain. But, what happens the brain can be reverted against us, without warning, or warning, with the primary aim to play all sorts of tricks against us, since various kinds of negative thoughts may occur.

The Most Oft-Repeated Negative Thoughts

Then, I will present an overview of the most frequently used negative thoughts and explain what each is made up of.

Negative thoughts, or unjustified assessments frequently come into our lives as we continually evaluate the circumstances that are likely to be presented to us. However, what we need to do is to evaluate ourselves in a reasonable way to ensure that they don't impact us more than is necessary and also be aware that their contents are not objective. This is why I want to identify the most prevalent negative thoughts that are likely to have occurred to you at one point or another throughout your lifetime:

1. Dichotomous thinking

Dichotomous thinking is a fixed and unflexible form of thinking that has no distinctions between black and white. It is therefore founded on the assumption that there are two distinct categories that are mutually exclusive and ignores the interrelated elements as well as other nuances.

This is because it's about thoughts that lie at the extremes. Examples:

* "You are either with I or against me."

* "Either I'm good at it ou I'm not."

* "All or nothing."

* "Now or never."

2. Beware of what they might be saying

Who hasn't been on the street and thought about "what would they say"? This is especially true when we feel that we're not properly dressed or that we must talk in public. This is extremely negative for us, as we can't live in the shadows of the opinions of others.

Keep in mind that everyone makes mistakes and what's most important is how you feel about yourself. We often worry too much about what others think about ourselves, and in the end it's impossible to find out what other people are thinking about you, just that you believe you know the thoughts they've got in their minds. This is a cognitive distortion, also known as thought reading.

For instance: "If I talk to them, I will say in a sloppy manner, I'll be a fool and they will be able to reject me."

3. Doing everything to ensure that everything is under control

When we are convinced that something could be wrong, our thoughts will agree with this notion and will suggest we quit the project. We will think of things like:

* "It certain that it will be wrong."

* "I'm not the best in this."

* "It's not worth it."

It is common to have ideas that all they can do is we remain in our familiar zone. But keep in mind that whoever "does not take risks, will not succeed. " Thoughts that are negative could cause us to not be able to leave the comfort of our homes.

4. Generalize the negative

A few people prefer to stick with negatives. This is why it's normal for people to believe that if someone is hurt they think that it will be an accepted norm. The path to success is often paved with many unsuccessful experiences. It is not a guarantee that nothing bad will ever occur because it only happened once is not a valid argument.

The tendency to generalize things is among the most common mistakes we make. It is important to be positive about your life. And when something happens for you, the next day is an entirely different day, however it won't be the case for you each day.

We fear negative outcomes and our predisposition means that we confirm what we were afraid of. For instance:

* Predictions: "If I speak in the public, I'll stumble."

* Perform the action with the premonitory thoughts and fear: "I begin to speak and, in fact like I was afraid I'm speaking in a stutter."

* Lastly, my mental assessment or conclusion is: "As I was afraid I've fallen off the track. It is recommended not to repeat the same speech in public" (avoidance).

5. We are disqualified as well as the remainder

If we are in disagreement with ourselves or any other person in our lives it is normal for thoughts that are not rational to come up in our minds for example:

170

1. "This person is not worth anything."

2. "But what you are claiming."

3. "I really love you."

However, it is important not to be swept away by emotion or insanity, because it can lead to quick conclusions that, in the future we might regret later.

6. The situation can be made more dramatic

Who hasn't thought "what could happen to my life" or "I will never meet someone similar to me" after enduring a relationship break-up? If we are looking to get over the challenges, it's recommended not to overstate everything and also to be prepared for the future. Many people have been through what you're going through (or more so) and all were able to get their lives back on track and get on with their lives. Negative thoughts are a result of the way you appear.

When we are confronted with everyday situations or symptoms that are normal, we can experience devastating effects, leading to great anxiety that, if not addressed correctly, could affect our lives.

It's great to believe that we are able to achieve anything and can reach the final destination. But one thing should be made evident the fact that there are times when this could be a challenge for us as a result of not meeting these expectations, we may cause a great deal of despair or stress.

Learn from Experimentation

Jim is a social anxiety sufferer. He is usually in his home and never is out due to his anxiety, even though Jim would like to go out and get to know people.

A friend of his invited Jim to dinner on a Saturday evening with several people, the majority of whom were not known to Jim. It was a challenging scenario for him to handle, typically it would be a no-go but this time, he decided to make it an opportunity to challenge himself personally and take the trip. The first thing he noticed was anxiety and negative thoughts as well as the desire to leave. But he gathered his strength and left before and after dinner. trying to "answer" the negative thoughts and to think rationally.

His thoughts included:

* Negative Thought that I'll be disqualified. They'll say I'm crazy. It's best to be at home/indiscriminate inference.

* Negative thought: I'm useless, I don't know how to be with people/classification

* Negative Thinking: Everyone will be watching me, and thinking negatively of me or reading my mind.

Negative Thinking: No one likes me/overgeneralization

I'm sorry, but Negative Thoughts Will Not Dissipate

Being conscious that negative thought patterns are present and analysing them objectively is the initial step. It is possible to give them the importance they deserve, but it's not going to remove the thoughts! It won't succeed in making us "think positively".

* Jim continues to feel unsecure in social settings, even though he is aware that his beliefs are unfounded but it's normal for him to feel that he has this feeling.

It's a fact that affects every one of us or has it been a reality for us? We know that negative thoughts are excessive or unfounded. Yet, even if we do we can't eliminate the thought.

In many instances I have had that negative thought although exaggerated or causing me to feel a lot of pain, may be partially true.

I will give the following example to you:

* Imagine that I've been suffering from headaches for several days and, within my head I start to think about the possibility that it might be something serious. I might even begin looking at the Internet... and convince myself that it's probably an endocrine tumor. The thought causes a lot of anxiety and a mental picture where I suddenly die in the course of a few months.

If I "try to avoid thinking" about the negative film and I try to keep it out of my mind, I'm likely not to achieve my goal, and the typical result is that it keeps me distracted for a time and then the fear comes back (maybe more intensely). It's also likely that I'm able to see rationally I'm exaggerating; however, I'm not able of stopping thinking about it.

If we examine this negative idea: "I'm sure it's a brain tumor and I'm likely to die" we can tell that this is untrue because it's exaggerated, and it considers the most dangerous of alternatives as a given ... however, it's impossible to say it's true because I'm not certain. It could be an actual brain tumor.

The problem is that it could be something important or not. That issue is just one possibility. It may be a tumor and it might be tension headache. I'm not sure.

If I think to myself "I'm exaggerating It's certainly not true!" It's just one option that I have, and so a portion of me is thinking. "Okay maybe it's something, but what do you do if it's true?" Then I'm hooked once more. It's back to the beginning.

The Thought Process influences action: Negativity calls for more Negativity

If we believe that something might be wrong, it's evident that it is likely to fail. This is referred to as self-fulfilling prophecy. What happens won't be the result of luck or fate as some claim instead of the negative energy that takes over our thoughts and affects our capacity to actions. This will cause an unintended chain reaction with devastating effects on the self-esteem of ours.

As per Beck (1983) Beck (1983), negative thoughts are rigid, rigid, and rigid and absolute. They also take the version of "I must", "I must think of". However positive thoughts are flexible, conceivable and adaptable. They are also able to take the format in the form of "I would like to", "I would like it to" or "I would like."

The day-to-day brains store every thought that occurs throughout the day, and prevents it from being processed within the brain's memory storage. Each day we experience 10,000 thoughts out of which 50,000 are negative. There are instances when certain thoughts could cause us into dilemma of whether they're good or not and if we don't recognize how to challenge them they could cause us to suffer harm.

When we begin to experience negative thoughts regarding the same issue, these could end up hurting us, as they become larger and more adolescent in the same time we are more convinced of them.

Every negative thought can drain our energy and rob us of all the vitality and strength we are blessed with from the moment we wake up until the time the time we fall asleep.

The more I repeat those negative ideas, they grow more powerful, gaining a foothold into our mental habits and making it more difficult to stay away from them.

Sometimes negative thoughts can be harmful the most, to the point that they could affect your lifestyle and character. Because in the end, the thoughts we think about, if don't know how to confront them, could harm our sense of value for our self-worth (self-esteem) or lead us to believe that innocent circumstances or signs are an imminent threat.

Why do we perpetuate negative thoughts if it actually causes us harm?

It could be described as the beginning of this is that the first negative thoughts start to afflict us. If we don't know how to handle these thoughts, they will end in reshaping our minds.

There are ways to get rid of this risky brain network. Neuroplasticity that we understand more and more, demonstrates that the brain can be fickle that we all have the ability to rid ourselves of ANTs and place positive thoughts to replace them. However, to achieve this the first thing to recognize is and realize that these are thoughts that we're not accountable (at at least not conscious).

Revealing Our True Critic

The reason for most discomfort are anti-neurotics, but they aren't often obvious. To recognize them it is important to know what the three major features these thoughts possess:

* They are messages that are specific to the individual.

The ant species usually have a distinct and frequent form, easily discernible in our speech. Since Jiminy Cricket speaks the same manner it is simple to recognize the ant. It is generally believed that these are messages that look like to be a shorthand brief phrase that pops up repeatedly in our heads over and again, taking the form of assumptions, memories or self-reproaches. Examples include the reconstruction of a previous moment ("if I'd done X and X, there would be no present X") and the creation of a fictional future incident ("I always make mistakes X but in the next it will repeat itself") or a guilt-based request (" I ought to have done X I should have done X. ").

* They are trustworthy messages

They appear spontaneously, automatically and suddenly appear in the mind, and without us making any prior judgement of the circumstances. Yet, despite their lack of solidity these arguments, they take these as absolute facts as concepts we've thought about for quite a while which is where the danger is in the assumption that we can believe that something is true, but it isn't.

If we can recognize these thoughts and examine them in a cold manner and objectively, we'll be able recognize the absurdity often.

While ANT from afar might seem absurd but the person suffering them believes that they are real and reliable, primarily because they aren't able to think about their implications (hence the good thing is sharing these with other people). We accept them as valid and unquestioningly, since they are believed to be true and spontaneous, something that is solvable by learning to examine their logic to determine if their claims aren't exaggerated.

* They are messages that do not have any thought.

To be able to control those negative thoughts in check (ending them in complete isolation isn't possible) We must recognize the voice in our head gives us only one perspective The ANTs are a response to the automated brain, which doesn't have a prior reflection of the brain. The judgment is made, however it seems the most rational. If we are able to identify these thoughts, and look at them in a detached manner and with carefulness, we'll be able to see the absurdity of them in the majority of instances and will be able to dispel these thoughts.

the Chain Negative of Thoughts

It is crucial to know why we're in the midst of negativity. There's a chain, the stimulus that triggers us to respond to the stimulus in a certain manner. Below, I've provided a few of the most typical examples that can aid in understanding the underlying causes with negative thinking, broadly:

* "Tomorrow I'm going to miss the meeting"

What do I think is the biggest concern about this meeting? Not having prepared the topic enough. What's the first challenge I have to deal with in my company? Do I have this thought whenever I'm under pressure?

What ever the answer is may be, I will not be able to predict the outcome until it occurs. Being anxious means suffering twice, first when you assume that the meeting could fail, and the second time if it does happen at all. What happens if everything goes smoothly?

We've wasted our time on discomfort that is not needed.

* "You surely think I'm an idiot"

As human beings who are social as we are, it's natural to be aware of the impression or opinion we leave on others however, deciding to act by examining what other people consider to be a loss regardless of the actions we take. We are not in control of what other

The same thing occurs to us when we are proud of our accomplishments. If we take away from our accomplishments We are inflicting ourselves a lot of pain. We don't need to wait until big occasions to examine our own performance.

* "I must be able to"

The phrases that begin with the words I must or have to are not typically the best chance of success. When we make use of these kinds of phrases, we're increasing the pressure of the actions we wish to take by feeling guilty for not doing it. The meaning of the word "requirement" decreases by replacing this by "I wish to".

These are only strokes in the vast array of subtleties and possibilities that occur in every circumstance that we face that is why it is crucial to understand what is happening to us in order to not harm ourselves by focusing on what we believe to be.

Conclusion

Dopamine is among the most frequently discussed neurotransmitters and all hormones nowadays. It's not surprising however, the more we learn about this, the greater issues are raised, and more possibilities are discovered that it impacts our lives on a daily basis.

It is fascinating is that, just like other chemicals, dopamine is one of the many ways in which the level of dopamine within the human body could increase. Certain of them could be considered to be natural, such as eating and exercising, whereas others can be achieved through more informal terms, less different drugs, medications and pharmacological supplements appear to produce the same result at first glance.

When you scratch the surface, it's not just important to increase your levels of dopamine to improve your quality of life in many ways - the most important thing is maintaining it and to keep it at a healthy level. Dopamine levels that are excessively high can damage one's nerve system, as well as no dopamine even. The results can vary in both cases however the end result is quite similar and all of it comes down with the notion that moderation is key.

This book should have provided you with information about the advantages of a healthy dopamine level and the dangers and risks of unhealthy levels. Additionally we hope that we provide you with useful tips on how to attain and maintain these levels while staying clear of any problems that are caused by the latter.